THE REAL MEAL REVOLUTION

www.realmealrevolution.com

Download the app

rmr.link/app

D1393072

WE'RE NOT EATING WHAT
WE'RE SUPPOSED TO EAT

★ ★ ★ ★ ★

AND THAT IS WHY
WE'RE GETTING FAT

THE ★REAL MEAL REVOLUTION

THE RADICAL, SUSTAINABLE
APPROACH TO HEALTHY EATING

PROFESSOR TIM NOAKES, JONNO PROUDFOOT AND SALLY-ANN CREED

ROBINSON

ROBINSON

First published in Great Britain in 2015 by Robinson

A CIP catalogue record for this book is available from the British Library.

ISBN: 978-1-47213-569-8 (paperback)

ISBN: 978-1-47213-570-4 (ebook)

Typeset in FF Unit

Desiged by Andrew Barron @ Thextension

Printed and bound in China

Robinson is an imprint of Constable & Robinson Ltd Carmelite House 50 Victoria Embankment London EC4Y 0DZ

An Hachette UK Company

www.hachette.co.uk

www.littlebrown.co.uk

The recommendations given in this book are solely intended as education and information and should not be taken as medical advice.

CONTENTS

THERE IS A WIDESPREAD MISCONCEPTION
THAT EATING FAT IS BAD FOR YOU ... THAT IT
IS A PRIMARY CAUSE OF HIGH BLOOD
PRESSURE, HEART DISEASE AND OBESITY.

★ ★ ★ ★ ★

REAL MEAL REVOLUTION IS FOCUSED ON
DEBUNKING THIS 'BIG FAT LIE' AND
RETURNING US TO A TIME WHEN THE HUMAN
RACE UNDERSTOOD THE IMPORTANCE OF REAL
FAT IN OUR DIETS.

INTRODUCTION

For a long time, human beings have been consumed by what we consume.
Our diets have been observed, studied and scrutinized while we attempt to balance our enjoyment of food with how to optimize our health.

We are clearly getting it wrong.

Obesity and diabetes are rapidly on the rise and those of us who are not obviously afflicted are becoming far too comfortable with our own slowly deteriorating health.

We tell ourselves that gaining weight, becoming slower and feeling weaker are a part of getting older and we resign ourselves to the way it is. On occasion some of us might experiment with extreme, quick-fix diets. But these are short-term solutions. We binge, we purge, but inevitably we return to our normal lives and our deteriorating physical states.

The Real Meal Revolution is for those of us who refuse to be satisfied with this status quo. It is both a startling revelation, and as old as humanity itself. It is not another diet that you can't sustain or a fad waiting to be forgotten, but a return to the way human beings are supposed to eat. It is informed by how our ancestors used to eat.

The work of a scientist, a nutritionist and a phenomenal chef, it turns their extensive research and experience into the definitive eating guide. This book combines undeniable scientific evidence, historical fact and mouth-watering recipes in one grand ambition:

To change the world, one meal at a time.

ABOUT THE AUTHORS

The Scientist
Professor Tim Noakes

Tim is a highly respected South African Professor of Exercise and Sports Science at the University of Cape Town. He has run more than seventy marathons and ultra-marathons and is the author of the books *The Lore of Running*, *Challenging Beliefs* and *Waterlogged*.

After publishing his latest book, Tim entered the dietary sphere, challenging the science behind obesity, coronary heart disease and heart attacks.

Subsequently he has dedicated his life to opening people's eyes to the myth of low-fat eating and the nutritional and environmental crisis it has now left us in. In this book, Tim unleashes the science behind the research and studies he has been conducting since the inception of this 'bee in his bonnet'.

The Nutritionist
Sally-Ann Creed

Sally-Ann spent most of her life sick with chronic asthma, sinusitis and panic disorder, undergoing many operations on her sinuses, and spending thirteen long years as a 'victim' of panic disorder and agoraphobia.

Through an adjustment in her diet, she has regained her health and qualified as a Nutritional Therapist (Post Graduate Diploma in Clinical Nutrition, Australia).
Her goal is to help others experience the same results.

Having found that food and supplements could dramatically change her life, giving her the quality of life she'd always dreamed about, Sally-Ann decided to study so that she could help others. Her story is relayed in her best-selling book *Let Food Be Your Medicine* – an easy-to-understand guide to healthy living.

The Chef
Jonno Proudfoot

After training and working in a five-times rated Top 10 restaurant in his early career, Jonno moved through a variety of food and wine establishments before finding his passion in Paleo and LCHF (low-carb, high-fat) cookery.

Since the birth of his interest in performance food and nutrition he has co-hosted 52 episodes of the award-winning South African children's cooking show *What's Your Flava*. He also starred in the reality cooking series *Ultimate Braai Master* in 2013.

On 23 March 2014, Jonno and his friend Thane Williams became the first two humans in history to swim from Mozambique to Madagascar. They swam 460 km in 24 days and set a world record for the longest open ocean unassisted stage swim of all time.

THE SOUTH AFRICAN EXPERIMENT

In March 2012, multi-award winning scientist Professor Tim Noakes discussed his own low-carbohydrate diet in an essay for an online news site. Noakes had managed to revive his health and his running career with an eating plan he claimed was also responsible for saving his life.

There was widespread public interest, not least because he had previously been a vocal advocate of the low-fat, high-carb diet. As one of the world's pre-eminent exercise science experts, this about-turn immediately caught the attention of the media. It also caught the attention of Kate Proudfoot, a Cape Town-based chef who followed Noakes' plan and proceeded to lose 20 kilograms (44 lbs) in less than six months.

Kate and her husband Jonno had just finished second in *Ultimate Braai Master* (a popular South African reality cooking show) and Jonno was preparing for another challenge; a 24-day, 459-kilometre (285-mile) swim from Mozambique to Madagascar in aid of the 'Miles for Smiles' charity managed by fellow South African adventurer and chef, David Grier.

Also a chef, with a passion for sports nutrition, Jonno decided to write a recipe book detailing his diet while he trained for this epic endurance feat. After seeing the results his wife was enjoying, he began to pay closer attention to Professor Noakes' advice.

When Noakes tweeted about Sally-Ann Creed being South Africa's premier Paleo (a diet designed to emulate the wild, raw foods eaten by humans during the Palaeolithic period) nutritionist, Jonno called her to arrange a meeting. It didn't take long before they were in a room discussing what was to become *The Real Meal Revolution*.

Noakes' initial commitment to write a 5,000-word introduction soon fell by the wayside. Instead, a few weeks after their first meeting he returned with a 20,000-word paper of overwhelmingly compelling scientific evidence. This exceptional body of work represented the past and present state of human nutrition, while providing a road map for the future.

Sally-Ann Creed then created an outline for an updated low-carb, high-fat eating plan, with all the advice and practical support that real people need to sustain a healthy life.

Finally, Jonno Proudfoot, with help from chef and extreme adventurer David Grier, turned the science and the blueprint into an unrivalled collection of delicious new recipes.

High demand was expected for what South Africans regarded as a practical guide to Tim Noakes' eating plan, but the extent of it could never have been anticipated. The first edition was released on 19 November 2013 and sold out on the same day. As fast as the book was printed, it was sold. There were no copies available in the month leading up to Christmas, and shortages across the country continued until the printing rate they finally caught up in May 2014.

The Real Meal Revolution sold over 160,000 copies in South Africa in its first six months. It was the top-selling book in the country for twenty-two weeks (at the time of writing) and was awarded the South African Book of the Year prize at the Nielsen Booksellers' Choice Awards 2014.

Welcome to the revolution!

WE ARE LED TO BELIEVE THAT WE ARE LAZY, THAT WE EAT TOO MUCH AND DON'T EXERCISE ENOUGH.

★ ★ ★ ★ ★

THESE ARE NOT THE CAUSE OF OUR HEALTH PROBLEMS. THEY ARE THE SYMPTOMS.

EATEN A STICK OF BAMBOO LATELY?

It's not likely that you spend much time thinking about the eating habits of bears. Granted, you probably see no reason to, but consider the diets of the koala, the panda and the polar bear. The koala bear lives solely on eucalyptus leaves; pandas eat only shoots and bamboo leaves while polar bears eat seals.

These three mammals have many biological similarities, yet they have very specific and unique dietary requirements. Their requirements could hardly be more different. And if they were fed on anything other than what they naturally eat, they would soon die.

The reason for this is obvious: all of the earth's creatures must eat the foods they were designed to eat. This 'design' depends on the nature of their creation or evolution (irrespective of which you believe).

Human beings are no different. As omnivores, we are certainly more complex than the average mammal, but our diet is unique and 'designed' for our species.

So if we want to know what foods are best for modern humans, we need to take a close look at what our ancestors ate before more recent (and radical) changes in our dietary options. We also need to look at what changes have occurred in recent years, and why they have taken place.

A BRIEF HISTORY OF THE HUMAN DIET

Although the Stone Age occurred literally 'ages' ago, today's most respected biologists, geneticists, paleoanthropologists and theorists believe that human genes have changed little since human beings began their journey on earth.

Approximately 200,000 years ago, early humans were hunter-gatherers. With limited resources at their disposal, prehistoric human beings could survive in very few places on earth. They hunted wild animals for fat and protein while their staples consisted of fruits and vegetables gathered from above and below the ground.

These early humans did not consume the same high-energy cereal grains – rice, corn wheat, etc. – that form such a huge part of the modern human diet. While they might have been able to harvest grains, the work required to process them into digestible form was excessive. Instead they foraged for and prepared other wild plants with a fraction of the effort.

It was only approximately 12,000 years ago that human beings began growing and processing cereal grains for consumption, and this radically changed the course of human nutrition.

We know this period as the first Agricultural Revolution. It was also the first catastrophe to befall the human diet.

THE FIRST GREAT DIETARY DISASTER

The Agricultural Revolution

It seemed like a good idea at the time ...

As the Ice Age began to thaw and humans moved north in search of new land, our species gradually developed, learnt a few handy new skills and transformed from hunter-gatherers into farmers.

You can almost imagine them, wandering in search of food one harsh winter, until a particularly angry chap decided he'd had enough of being tired and hungry. 'There has to be an easier way!'(he may or may not have exclaimed), and not long after that human beings had figured out how to harvest crops and domesticate animals.

Suddenly there was no incentive to roam around in search of food. They could stay put and concentrate their energy on building settlements, making babies, cultivating crops and storing food for a rainy day.

Eventually this shift from a nomadic to a sedentary society brought with it many other innovations. From specialization and division of labour to trading economies, this 'revolution' resulted in civilization as we know it. And although it did wonders for human development, it produced a diet that – it turns out – was far less civilized. For with this switch to a grain-based diet humans became smaller, fatter and more sickly with an average life expectancy that dropped from 40 to about 20 years. In fact, only in the last century have humans regained the same heights that we enjoyed 12,000 years ago. The only advantage that we gained from this new diet was greater reproductive success. Indeed, the agricultural revolution was the direct cause of the subsequent over-population of planet earth.

Which brings us back to grains and cereals. The ability to cultivate crops meant that our ancestors soon developed techniques to turn these hard, dry seeds into various forms that our bodies can digest. This was an important breakthrough because dry grains are more durable and abundant than other staple 'foods'. They became valuable because they could be produced with minimum effort, stored for longer, and when all was said and done, could be traded for just about anything.

Fast forward to today, and after a few thousand years of agricultural innovations we have learnt not only how to harvest these grains, but also how to process and refine them to the point where they offer us little of what we need and a whole lot of what we don't.

It's astounding how much human health has deteriorated since we moved away from fat and protein and towards a diet of processed, carbohydrate-based foods. And while we have mainly human endeavour and good intentions to thank for this, the second great disaster can be blamed on political forces and the brazen distortion of scientific fact.

For more details, please turn to pages 246–91.

HUMAN BEINGS HAVE ONLY BEEN EATING
REFINED CARBS FOR THE LAST 100 YEARS,

★★★★★

OR LESS THAN 1 PER CENT OF
OUR EXISTENCE.

THE SECOND PUNCH TO THE GUT

The 1977 Dietary Goal for Americans

The US Senate produced the dietary outline that is still relied on today – but the science was flawed.

In 1953, the American biochemist Ancel Keys (PhD) published a study purporting to show the relationship between the amount of fat in the diet, the level of cholesterol and the risk of heart attack.

His conclusion was essentially that the fat in our diets increases our blood cholesterol levels, thereby clogging our arteries and directly resulting in heart disease.

But there were a number of problems with Keys' science. For starters, of the twenty-two countries in the study, he decided to ignore sixteen of them and use data from the six that best supported his theory. He also chose not to factor in the massive growth in cigarette smoking beginning after World War I that coincided with a sudden rise in heart disease which happened at the same time. Furthermore, Keys was an academic theorist who never actually treated a patient suffering from heart disease.

These factors, along with his failure to prove causality through randomized clinical trials – a fundamental requirement – put his findings seriously into question.

But despite these numerous shortcomings, criticism and warnings from respected professionals, the 1977 US Senate Select Committee on Nutrition and Human Needs used Keys' study as the basis for their dietary recommendations.

The resulting high-carb, low-fat (HCLF) diet which the guidelines promoted has since been adopted throughout most of the Western world. It has much to answer for – in particular the dramatic rise in global rates of obesity and diabetes since 1980.

For more details, please turn to pages 246–91.

THE THIRD BODY BLOW

Genetically Modified Foods

Commercial profitability – and not your health – is what drives the food industry.

For the last few decades, the cereal and grains that (regrettably) constitute a large part of our diets have started taking on an even more deceptive form.

The chemical composition of an increasing number of crops is being altered using genetic engineering. The purpose of this is to introduce something to the crop that does not occur naturally, to improve its life span, taste or resistance to pesticides.

GM crops might look familiar, but their genetic makeup is not. These fruits and veggies end up with far higher sugar and carbohydrate quantities than their natural cousins.

Today, more than 12 per cent of the world's crops are genetically modified. This number increases every day because the powerful commercial and political influences have concluded that they offer no greater risk to our health than natural foods. However, what is overlooked is that human biology has adapted to the meats, fruits and vegetables our ancestors have consumed since antiquity.

So in the long history of human existence, cereal grains are a brand new development. We have included them in our diets for a fraction of human existence. Throw a mere twenty years of genetically modified foods into the mix, and our poor bodies get even more confused. Worse, we have no idea what will be the effects of these recent changes on the long-term health of humans.

Like the koala, panda or polar bear, human beings have a naturally prescribed diet that we followed diligently for hundreds of thousands, perhaps millions, of years. But unlike the other mammals, who without thought continue to eat that for which they are designed, we have recently lost our way.

For more details, please turn to pages 246–91.

THE ORIGIN OF BANTING

We owe it to William, William and William

(not to mention Wilhelm)

As we've discovered, our ancestors deserve the credit for developing the low-carb, high-fat (LCHF) movement. It was the only diet they knew, and they followed it without any fanfare until commerical enterprise took over.

But after they lost their way, a London undertaker named William Banting rediscovered LCHF eating. By 1862, the obese Mr Banting had packed on quite enough weight and was desperate to lose it. His doctor, William Harvey, went out on a limb, but restricted the amount of carbohydrates that Mr Banting could eat.

Harvey had recently attended a series of lectures delivered by the iconic French physiologist Claude Bernard, who had just discovered that the liver produces glucose. For reasons that remain uncertain, Harvey concluded from this that limiting carbohydrates and sugars would benefit obese and diabetic patients. His advice to Banting was simple:

★ Eat four moderate meals a day, instead of three large meals

★ Do not consume bread, milk, butter, beer, sugar or potatoes
   (it was mistakenly believed that butter contained starch)

★ Avoid root crops like carrots, beetroot, turnip and parsnips

★ Avoid 'farinaceous foods' (starchy foods including grains)

Banting's remarkable weight loss was big news after he published a book detailing his story, and in no time various iterations of the Harvey/Banting diet sparked up all over the world. Some of these suggested that it was more protein and less fat that was required; others focused on the consumption of fat as being key; but they all agreed that carbohydrates should be kept to a minimum.

With William Banting taking a back seat, it was a German physician, Dr Wilhelm Ebstein, who now carried the torch for the original LCHF version as it began to spread throughout Europe.

In the United States in 1892, Dr William Osler prescribed the high-fat version of the diet as the definitive treatment for obesity. As a founding professor of the iconic Johns Hopkins Hospital and a man described as 'the father of modern medicine', he added a great deal of weight to the movement (if you'll pardon the expression).

Banting was the standard treatment for weight loss in all major European and North American medical schools until the end of World War II, when it was excluded from all the major medical and nutritional textbooks. It was replaced with its polar opposite, the currently popular low-fat, high-carb diet. This change would have disastrous consequences for human health over the next six decades. In addition, since the 1950s, significant political, commercial and other pressures have influenced advice on what is a healthy diet. A good example of this involves one of the more popular advocates of the movement and one of the more controversial United States Presidents.

Dr Robert Atkins published his *Diet Revolution* in 1972, around the same time that President Richard Nixon was gearing up for re-election. Atkins' book promoted the idea that carbohydrates – not fat – are the cause of the obesity epidemic so that dietary carbohydrates – not fats – should be restricted. This ran quite contrary to the direction in which US politics was driving dietary advice. The key election strategy demands that you keep your voters happy. In Nixon's case, it meant satisfying US farmers and consumers at the same time. Nixon's Secretary of Agriculture, Earl Butz, did this by industrializing the production of maize and soy, thereby keeping prices low and profits high. The demand for grain soared.

This was clearly not the time for Atkins to challenge the status quo. In 1977 the United States Senate Committee released the high-carb, low-fat Dietary Goal for Americans, and the rest is history.

THANKS FOR NOTHING, CARBS

There are three macronutrients in the human diet – protein, fats and carbohydrates. Two of these are essential for our survival, but the third is completely unnecessary. It may come as a big surprise to you that carbohydrate is the only macronutrient we don't need.

Carbohydrates can do only one of two things for us. They can either be burned as fuel or stored in the body, either as carbohydrate in the liver and muscles, or as fat in the liver and fat (adipose) tissues. There is no other option. Fats and protein, on the other hand, are important for building, developing and maintaining the body's structures. In addition both fat and protein can be used as energy sources in the body.

Every gram of carbohydrate that we consume must be burnt immediately, as a fuel, or it will be stored either as fat or glycogen (a complex form of glucose). The problem is that, because of our genetic makeup, all humans have a different degree of insulin resistance (IR). And the more severe the insulin resistance, the more difficulty the body has in processessing carbohydrates. As a result, high carbohydrate diets eaten for decades by those with insulin resistance will inevitably lead to ill-heath – the metabolic syndrome, obesity and diabetes.

1 Eating carbs causes your blood glucose to rise.

2 Insulin is secreted by your pancreas to bring down your blood glucose level.

3 If you can't burn the carbohydrate immediately, the liver turns it into fat (leading to fatty liver) or sends it to be stored in fat cells (as fat).

4 The carbohydrates do not satisfy hunger – they stimulate it. So the insulin-resistant person eating a high-carb diet is perpetually hungry. And because of the addictive nature of sugar and carbohydrates, the hungry will always make the same addictive food choices that cause the problem in the first place.

5 Repeating this process five or more times a day for decades leaves us sick and unhealthy with the metabolic syndrome.

The more insulin resistant we are, the more damaging carbohydrates will be, leaving us more susceptible to obesity, diabetes, high blood pressure and heart disease.

The obesity epidemic began with people eating far more energy in the form of carbohydrates, because they are always hungry. As soon as you cut carbohydrates out, that constant hunger disappears.

Hungry?

'Won't I be starving without carbs?' This is a common question and an understandable one. The short answer is 'no'. There is no hunger when you ditch carbs because you are encouraged to listen to your body and eat as much as you need.

The longer answer explains how this is possible. There is a vital component of your brain called an appestat. The function of this essential mechanism is to regulate your appetite. However, if you have a carb-rich diet, there's every chance that your appestat has been hijacked by the allure of all those addictive foods and isn't doing what it's supposed to.

This is because carbs have the devastating ability to give you nothing but hunger. Bereft of nutrients and packed with salt and sugar, they just make you want more. Think about it in terms of your favourite carb-based snacks. These sweet or salty little pretenders are incredibly addictive and don't make you feel full. Your body struggles to extract anything that it needs from these 'foods', so it's fooled into thinking it needs more.

TODAY'S DIETARY ADVICE ASSUMES THAT EVERYONE CAN EAT 6–11 SERVINGS OF GRAINS A DAY.

★ ★ ★ ★ ★

THIS IS SIMPLY NOT THE CASE.

In this case, your appestat isn't working. It's been tampered with, because most of the products in question are processed and developed with one purpose in mind: to make you want more. They are tested and refined to the point where they are as addictive as they are destructive. Scientists even have a name for this: they call it the 'bliss point'. This is the perfect combination of sugar, salt and fat in the engineered food that will entice you to eat as much of the product as you can. And want to come back for more. That is why it is impossible to eat one potato chip. The product is engineered to make you finish the packet. And then to search for a second.

Proteins and fats, on the other hand, are rich in nutrients. They make you feel full when you are full, which has so many positive effects on your health and your life. In effect, this addresses any food-related issues that you might face by tackling them at their root. When you aren't constantly hungry and thinking about your next meal, your mind is freed up to be more rational, relaxed and focused on something more productive.

The bottom line is, you shouldn't need to count calories. Our ancestors didn't and they never got fat. Your appestat has been fine-tuned for generations to ensure that you remain at your optimum weight. As long as your appestat is working and your body is listening, you can eat without guilt.

After adopting a low-carb, high-fat eating plan, you will soon notice that your cravings disappear. There is no binge eating because your body tells you everything you need to know.

THERE'S A BELIEF THAT EATING FAT WILL MAKE YOU FAT, BECAUSE IT'S FULL OF CALORIES.

★ ★ ★ ★ ★

IT'S COMPLETELY FALSE – BECAUSE IT FORGETS THAT YOU HAVE A BRAIN.

THE HEART OF THE MATTER

Another logical question that plagues many people who are considering a low-carb, high-fat diet involves the perceived danger of cholesterol and heart disease.

There is a longstanding misconception that fat 'causes cholesterol', and cholesterol causes heart disease. It comes from the falsely simplistic view that saturated fat in the diet is converted into cholesterol, which then clogs the arteries. This could not be further from the truth.

To begin with, cholesterol is not bad. Without cholesterol serving its multiple vital functions in our bodies, we would all be dead.

'Cholesterol' is not the problem, but *some* Lipoproteins are the problem. Let us explain.

Cholesterol is a fatty substance that is insoluble in water. To transport cholesterol in the blood from the liver (where it is produced) to the cells (where it is needed), it must be bound into a water-soluble protein-rich carrier. This is known as a lipoprotein. There are many different lipoproteins. Most are considered either harmless or protective against heart disease. Currently it is believed that the dangerous lipoprotein that damages our arteries is the small dense LDL-cholesterol particle. These particles are increased in those who eat high-carbohydrate diets and reduced in those replacing carbohydrate in their diets with more fat and protein.

If you are insulin resistant and you eat a high-carbohydrate diet, you are likely to damage the lining of your arteries by increasing the number of small, dense LDL-cholesterol particles that are circulating in your bloodstream. What's more, the frequent spikes in blood glucose and insulin concentrations irritate the arterial linings inducing a state of arterial inflammation. These inflamed arteries can then allow the entry of these small, dense, LDL-particles causing the arterial damage we call plaque accumulation that leads to atherosclerosis (hardening of the arteries).

Therefore it is biologically impossible for humans to convert dietary saturated fat into LDL cholesterol because that simply does not happen. The fat we eat in the diet is first stored as fat in our fat cells. Some of that fat is then returned to the bloodstream and in the liver, cholesterol, triglyceride and protein is added, producing the different lipoprotein fractions that then carry the cholesterol to the cells for their use.

Your cholesterol may well increase on a high-fat diet, *but this is not necessarily 'bad' as long as the increase is in the favourable lipoprotein fractions like HDL cholesterol and the large fluffy LDL particles*. What is bad is if the harmful lipoproteins, especially the small dense LDL cholesterol particles, increase. And this is much more likely to occur on a high-carbohydrate diet in those with insulin resistance.

Professor Noakes explains this in more detail on pages 246–91.

THE BANTING MANIFESTO
WHAT IS BANTING?

It is learning you are right to challenge your existing beliefs.

It is taking control of your life and living on your terms.

It is refusing to accept the status quo.

It is making healthy choices and knowing why.

It is being empowered, not overpowered by what you eat.

It is digging in. Not passing up.

Satisfying. Not depriving.

Eating. Not abstaining.

It is indulging. In delicious meals you used to think were harmful.

It is avoiding other meals you believed to be good.

It is overcoming your body's harmful addiction to sugars and carbs.

It is saying 'yes' to real fats and real foods, and 'no' to refined grains and processed goods.

It is challenging the not-so-supermarket machine.

It is voting against the foods you don't want by choosing the ones you do.

It is not a diet. It is a food revolution.

WHAT WILL BANTING DO FOR YOU?

Banting is not just for overweight people and diabetics. We can all benefit from following it.

There are different ways to apply the principles, and some people can handle carbohydrates better than others. The main thrust of the Banting proposition, however, is limiting carbohydrates while eliminating both sugar and toxic seed oils.

By Banting, you can expect

★ More energy

★ Fewer (or no) cravings

★ No hunger

★ Weight loss

★ Better blood glucose and insulin readings

★ Enhanced athletic performance

★ Increased mental focus

★ Better sleeping habits

★ Much better health in every aspect

The list of benefits is extensive, but these are the most universally experienced. Professor Noakes has gone into great detail around Type 2 Diabetes as well as athletic performance while Banting from page 249. For more information on the benefits of Banting with various conditions such as polycystic ovary syndrome (PCOS); digestive conditions; allergies and cancer; during pregnancy, childhood and menopause, please visit our website.

Ours is a society built on constant eating – however when Banting, snacking becomes a thing of the past. After a while it is not unusual to find you are only eating one or two meals a day, yet without hunger between meals. Essentially you are looking to eat only when hungry. Stop when you feel full, and eat again when you feel hungry.

When you begin, you will probably need a week or two for the body to adapt – but once this is done the hunger and cravings disappear. You won't feel hungry or have to plan for sugar lows. Even Type 1 diabetics using insulin will benefit because by reducing their carbohydrate intakes they will need to use less insulin. And it is the insulin that causes blood-sugar lows. So the less insulin they need to inject, the less frequently they will develop low blood-sugar concentrations

Banting comprises mainly animal protein (including poultry, eggs and fish), saturated animal fats (including lard, duck fat and butter), coconut oil, olive oil and macadamia oil, some cheeses and dairy products, some nuts and seeds (if appropriate), fresh vegetables grown mostly above the ground and a few berries. There are no grains, seed oils or sugars (see the Green, Orange and Red Lists on pages 40–45 for more guidance).

The following basics apply to everyone in virtually every stage of one's life, and will lay the foundation for the various states that follow. It is imperative if you want to get the most of out of this programme that you follow the guidelines that follow.

★ Avoid all processed food, pre-packed, boxed, fast food, food in wrappers, etc.

★ Completely exclude all sugar, fructose, maltose, agave products – anything sugary

★ Eliminate all grain products (wheat, barley, spelt, oats, rye, corn, etc.) – this applies to the grain in its 'whole grain' form as well as its refined flour form

★ Replace all seed oils (canola, sunflower, safflower, cottonseed, grapeseed) and other inflammatory polyunsaturated oils (whether cold-pressed, extra-virgin or organic) with healthy saturated fats as outlined in this book, and be aware 99 per cent of prepared products will contain these damaged oils. Extra virgin olive oil and virgin coconut oil are encouraged freely

★ Eliminate all refined carbohydrates (see section on carbohydrates, pages 34–35), and if you wish to follow the plan where a few carbs are included, aim for those sourced from vegetables, not grains or sugars. If you find this difficult to begin with, aim for a little rye or oats, or perhaps some quinoa or buckwheat – but keep these to a minimum as you transition to the no-grain stage. This is an important part of the Banting plan

★ Aim for high-fat dairy products, not skimmed or reduced fat, 'lite' or fat-free alternatives – they must be full-fat. This is assuming you are not intolerant to dairy products, and find they do not affect your weight loss or blood-sugar levels

★ Avoid all soya products with the exception of a little MSG-free soy sauce now and then. Soya is a genetically modified, toxic non-food with a host of problems and should not be consumed by man or beast

★ A cup of homemade broth each day would be very helpful in terms of providing the extra minerals needed to alleviate cramping while supplying beneficial nutrients and quality liquid to the daily diet (see recipe on page 64).

Be Realistic

Of course there is always the odd occasion where it's impossible to dodge that piece of cheesecake, glass of sherry or lovingly made pasta Alfredo. But this is where you need to muster up all the willpower you have to indulge in a very small portion (and make sure it's taken after a protein-rich and/or fat-rich meal to buffer any sugar rush).

First prize goes to anyone who can avoid having any of these foods entirely. You'll discover very soon that your options aren't so limited as you might expect.

There are certain conditions and phases in life that require tweaking to the basics of Banting. We've run through these on pages 46–47 so you can tailor your Banting based on your own specific requirements.

PERHAPS THE BIGGEST ISSUE PEOPLE FACE IN TRYING TO FOLLOW THE HEALTHIEST POSSIBLE EATING PLAN

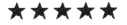

IS IDENTIFYING WHAT THAT PLAN IS.

BANTING EXPLAINED

WHERE TO BEGIN

There's a lot to learn, and a lot of delicious food to be eaten, so let's dive straight in. When you begin Banting, you will need to:

★ Toss out the offending foods and non-foods

★ Decide on what you would like to eat

★ Shop for the correct ingredients – have a look at the recipes and use as many of these as possible to make this a super-tasty experience. The recipes are all carefully designed to fit into the Banting lifestyle so using this book is safe in every aspect.

Start with your fridge. Is there anything that will tempt you to go off the rails? Clean the fridge out and prepare it for fresh produce.

Next, go to your kitchen cupboards and critically examine the tins of food, the bottles of sauce, dressings and pasta mixes – none of these will be suitable so donate them to a food bank or get rid of them altogether. Are there boxes of cereal, crisps and other 'rainy day' treats there? Get rid of them. All these foods have hidden carbs and sugars, and they will derail your best efforts. Do you have potatoes, crackers, pasta, rice or white flour in the cupboard? Say goodbye – it's a known fact that failing to plan is planning to fail.

Now you can go shopping. Choose the recipes from this book that you want to start with and make a list of all the fresh ingredients you will need. Don't buy too much so that you feel you have to eat it all before it goes off. Shopping every few days for fresh ingredients full of nutrients is preferable to having vegetables lose their appeal and nutrition, which may mean you will waste food and money when you inevitably throw them away.

By planning ahead from the recipes you won't have any wasted ingredients. It's a great idea to sit and plan a week or a few days at a time. Make additional portions of the foods you can freeze so that on busy days you can head to the freezer for a LCHF meal and just add a salad.

It helps to always have the following in your fridge for quick meals and snacks if necessary:

- ★ Roast chicken
- ★ Boiled eggs
- ★ Washed salad leaves
- ★ Sliced vegetables

- ★ Beef jerky and natural cured meats
- ★ Nuts and seeds
- ★ Fresh berries
- ★ Other healthy low-carb foods

Vegetables

Everyone can agree that vegetables are a valuable source of nutrition for the human body, even those who dislike them. Almost all permitted carbohydrates in the Banting lifestyle come from vegetables. They offer an enormous range of nutrients, some of which have not even yet been discovered. For example, just one cup of broccoli boasts a vitamin C level of 116 mg, 76 mcg folate, 456 mg potassium and 72 mg calcium. And that's not including the phytochemicals, the fibre or any of the other complex nutrients – all for under 5 g net carbs per cup. Cruciferous vegetables are powerful anti-carcinogens, and on this programme, leafy greens such as spinach, cabbage, Brussels sprouts and kale can all be eaten freely (you will find comprehensive lists of cruciferous vegetables on the Net). They are self-limiting; nobody gets 'addicted' to them or over-eats on these vegetables, so they are regarded as 'eat all you like' foods.

By steaming broccoli for just 90 seconds you will derive the most sulforaphane and indole-3-carbinol from it – two incredibly powerful anti-cancer agents. It's advisable to steam vegetables from the brassica family lightly as this renders the goitrogens present in these vegetables inactive. Goitrogens are responsible for depressing thyroid function in some people, so if your thyroid is underactive you don't want to eat a lot of raw broccoli, cauliflower and cabbage. Steaming allows you to not only get the best out of them, but to avoid the potential hypothyroid effect.

Brightly coloured vegetables 'advertise' their nutritional status and are powerhouses of important phytochemicals, antioxidants and nutrients which support eye health and brain health, mop up free radicals formed as by-products of living, provide fibre, give us extra liquid, taste delicious and, in the case of vegetables like garlic and onions, offer natural antibiotics and probiotics. Vegetables are undeniably an important part of any healthy diet. The fibre from plants is also responsible, together with intestinal bacteria, for the production of short-chain fatty acids (SCFA) which feed the walls of the intestine and protect against intestinal cancers.

Some vegetables deliver greater benefits when they are cooked than in their raw state. The carrot is a great example, and while this is a root vegetable that is limited on Banting due to its higher carb content, there are some interesting nutrients we can get from carrots. A substance called falcarinol found in carrots has been shown to reduce the risk of cancer, according to researchers at the Danish Institute of Agricultural Sciences (DIAS). Kirsten Brandt, head of the research department, commented that isolated cancer cells grow more slowly when exposed to falcarinol.

Tomatoes are very beneficial cooked, as only in their cooked form is the valuable lycopene able to be absorbed by the body as a protective measure against prostate cancer – and incidentally lycopene is only released in a cooked tomato in the presence of fat, so be generous with the fat when sautéing them. Garlic, both raw and cooked, contains sulphur, flavonoids and selenium – all potent anti-cancer agents, working mainly in the digestive tract and preventing organ cancers. It's said you can never have too much money, or too much garlic.

Onions are best cooked in oil to release their phytochemicals. Avoiding fat prevents the rich source of quercetin (a powerful antioxidant and antihistamine) from being released and absorbed, so cooking onions in fat rather than water is the best way to appreciate their health benefits. Onions are also good for normalizing blood viscosity and fighting infection. They have even been credited with helping to detoxify heavy metals like cadmium and arsenic from the body, which cause cancer due to the high levels of cysteine and methionine (amino acids) present. These amino acids are also present to a lesser extent in egg yolks. There is a fair amount of vitamin C to be found in onions, which is also known for detoxifying heavy metals.

Protein

Proteins are long complex chains of amino acids, needed for building and repairing our bodies. Excluding bone and water, the body is made up almost entirely of protein. The only readily available natural source of 'complete' proteins (those that contain all of the essential amino acids needed) are found in the animal kingdom and include seafood, poultry, eggs, beef, lamb, game and dairy products. Many other foods contain some protein, but only animal protein is 'complete' protein. Vegetarian protein is not complete, and various different food sources are needed to make up those amino acids. However, a vegetarian diet is by nature a carbohydrate-rich diet, and usually a very low-fat diet. You can clearly see the problem here for successful Banting if you are vegetarian.

Fat

Dietary fats are essential to life, and though much maligned in the past, they are pivotal to attaining permanent weight loss and glowing health. Some fats are not good for you, such as hydrogenated or partially hydrogenated fats (found in margarines and commercially baked and processed foods), all seed oils and trans fats (trans fats are damaged fats found in many margarines, seed oils and processed food).

All these unhealthy fats are high in omega-6 fatty acids, also extremely inflammatory, and vie for position in our receptor sites with the healthier omega-3 fatty acids. By taking in too many omega-6s, you sabotage the body's ability to make use of omega-3s, which are anti-inflammatory and health-promoting.

Better fats and oils to choose are those that are found in nature and these are more stable, such as any fat from animals like lard, duck fat and butter, as well as coconut oil, olive oil and macadamia nut oil. When cooking, saturated fat is superior to all other fats thanks to its stability. Healthy fat intake does not lead to fat storage, unless it is mixed with sugar and other carbohydrates. Fat functions well with protein and thus by avoiding high-carbohydrate foods, especially if refined, you will spare yourself the inflammation that accompanies this way of eating.

Carbohydrates

Carbs are virtually everything that is not fat or protein, and are made from long chains of carbon, hydrogen and oxygen atoms. All the sugars, including sucrose, fructose, glucose, etc. are known as simple carbohydrates, while complex carbohydrates are those we find in vegetables, fruit, nuts, seeds and grains. In fact you will find limited amounts of carbohydrates in almost all foods, other than pure fat or pure protein.

In the body even complex carbohydrates are converted to glucose, so keeping your carbohydrate intake low is important for success when Banting. The fibre content of carbohydrate-containing food is not digested, though, and becomes an ally when it comes to weight control.

The carbohydrate weight of a food might be 9 grams, with four of those being fibre, which would then mean the 'net carb count' of that food would be just 5 g. Fibre is valuable in its natural form (as found in vegetables and even meat) as it 'sweeps' the waste from the body, produces valuable short-chain fatty acids to feed the mucosa of the intestines, and is an important food source for the healthy bacterial cultures living in the digestive system.

The reason for the Banting obsession with cutting carbohydrates is because carbohydrates elicit an insulin response. Insulin by nature is both an inflammatory hormone and a fat-storing hormone, which we wish to keep as low as possible using only the barest minimum to remove the glucose from the bloodstream to turn it into energy. The excess is stored as fat, and this acts as a back-up fuel supply. The problem is that we seldom use up the stored fuel, and continue to eat far too much in the way of carbohydrates for the body to use immediately, so that the stored fat is never needed and instead continues to be built upon.

By keeping the body's level of glucose in a narrow range, you prevent the huge release of insulin that is usually required to clear the glucose from the blood after a high-carbohydrate meal. Stable blood sugar allows the body to begin to burn the stored fat as energy. Because besides being the fat-building hormone, insulin is also the hormone that prevents our bodies from burning all the fat stored in our fat cells. So if you want to start burning the fat that is stored in your fat cells, you *must* ensure that your insulin levels are as low as possible! And you can only do that by limiting carbs. And the more insulin resistant you are, the more you must restrict your carb intake.

Why soya, corn and MSG are not welcome

Soy/soya

Soy is *never* recommended by anyone who has a shred of scientific nutritional knowledge. It's a very poor source of protein and shouldn't be confused with 'real' animal protein. Soy should never be considered as an alternative source of protein. Soy beans are a very cheap crop to grow, and now globally over 95 per cent is genetically modified

(GMO). But even 'organic' soya contains toxic phytochemicals and has an extensive list of problems associated with its use, including:

★ Suppression of thyroid hormones (causing hypothyroid and goitres)

★ Digestive distress

★ Immune system breakdown

★ Severe allergies

★ ADD and ADHD

★ Higher risk of heart disease

★ Malnutrition (phytates present in soy prevent absorption of protein, calcium, magnesium, iron and zinc)

★ Contains very high levels of oestrogen which affects sperm (a Harvard study showed a correlation between soy intake and low sperm count)

★ Promotes fat storage

★ Soybean oil has been linked to cancer

★ Hexane (a constituent of petrol) is used in its manufacture

There are dozens of other reasons not to touch soy – but these should suffice.

Corn

Like soya, corn is virtually always GMO, which is bad enough, but corn is a very high-carbohydrate food too. The carb value also rises dramatically with each stage of the refining process; from coarse cornmeal to the finest flour or starch, corn comes in many forms. It is also one of those ubiquitous products which, like soy, have invaded every kind of processed food. A poor source of nutrients, in the spirit of what we aim to share with you in this book we suggest you avoid corn entirely.

Monosodium Glutamate (MSG)

The American neurosurgeon Dr Russell Blaylock is one of the experts in the dangers of MSG. His research has found that the cells of the brain literally 'excite themselves to death' in the presence of MSG. It is a taste enhancer and is found as dozens of aliases, one of the most common being 'textured vegetable protein'. An exceptionally toxic substance, it has no place in anyone's diet – eating real, non-processed food will be your best protection against MSG, as it is added to almost all processed food to improve taste.

Fermented foods

Fermenting food is a lost art – a practice used to keep the digestive and immune systems healthy, as the digestive system makes up 70 per cent of the body's entire immune system. A healthy balance of good and bad bacteria needs to be maintained for optimal health. The gut is known as the 'second brain' and contains more neurotransmitters than the brain itself.

Diet plays a key role in keeping the gut healthy, and fermented foods in the diet are the perfect way to replenish healthy gut bacteria. They provide the body with a natural source of probiotics. Traditional cultures from the beginning of time have all eaten fermented foods, even though they may not have understood their complexity or role in the body. For many hundreds of years there were no refrigerators so fermenting was a wonderful way to preserve food as well as to provide healing properties for the body. The process enhances nutrient content with beneficial microbes and enzymes, and valuable vitamin K2 is provided to the body, which may prevent heart disease and osteoporosis.

Lacto-fermentation involves plunging vegetables into salt-water brine that kills any unwanted microbes, allowing the beneficial bacteria to proliferate. A chemical reaction then occurs causing *lactobacilli* to break down the starches and sugars of the vegetable and produce lactic acid, preserving the vegetables. A nutrient-dense food is created which is highly therapeutic when eaten in small amounts, adding a few spoons to one's food daily. Fermented foods nourish, balance and help to heal the gut and enhance immunity.

Stevia, sugar alcohols and artificial sweeteners

These are very helpful in the interim stage of switching suddenly from a sugary diet to a no-sugar diet. This can be extremely difficult for some people, and while the ideal is to retrain your tastebuds away from the desire for sugar, realistically this is only going to happen for a very few people. If a sugar alcohol or natural sweetener such as stevia helps you to avoid resorting to sugar or artificial sweeteners, it is worth using them. The other thing about some sugar alcohols is that with their low or zero carb count, they can be used to bring flavour to some foods.

Stevia is a natural herb, and has been shown to have blood-sugar balancing benefits. It contains no calories, no carbs and is 600 times sweeter than sugar, so just a tiny bit of powder or liquid is used in sweetening a beverage or dish. This would be our sweetener of choice, but one could also use a sugar alcohol such as erythritol or xylitol for bulk in baking. These can be really helpful for those who struggle with sugar cravings, and can make the difference between staying on the plan and returning to a sugary diet. They taste almost identical to sugar, but are considerably more expensive.

Artificial sweeteners, on the other hand, are particularly harmful to the body and the brain, and amazingly – though often touted as 'slimming aids' – in fact have been shown to increase hunger and cause weight gain. There are many of these artificial sweeteners, including sucralose, acesulfame K, cyclamates, saccharine, etc. – all of which are bad for a variety of reasons. It's safe to say you will sabotage any attempt to improve your health and weight if you use these sweeteners. Make a clean break from sugar, or use stevia, xylitol or erythritol. The added benefit of sugar alcohols is that if you have too much (over nine teaspoons a day), you will have looser stools, which may actually help to combat a troublesome constipation problem in the early stages of the programme, but that's the worst that can happen. Stevia does not have this effect, and it has been shown to help to balance blood sugar.

Parting comments

1 Your weight on your bathroom scales is the best measure of whether your lower carbohydrate intake is also producing a lower calorie intake (according to the Yudkin Paradox). This is because the best measure of your daily caloric balance is what the scale tells you is your weight. If your weight is dropping, then your calorie intake is less than your intake. If your weight is stable, then your intake equals your expenditure. And if your weight is increasing, then your calorie intake exceeds your energy expenditure. There are of course some exceptions to this absolute rule. For example, if water is being lost or retained or if muscle is being added, then this rule is broken. But those are usually short-term effects – over weeks or months the bathroom scales are the most accurate measure of whether or not Banting has produced a change in the number of calories you are eating daily.

2 While Banting produces spectacular results in a majority of people who follow it and who are able to reduce their carbohydrate intakes to very low values, there are some, more commonly women, in whom the results are less spectacular. This may be because they are particularly sensitive to protein and perhaps secrete excessive amounts of insulin in response to protein ingestion. One option is to reduce the protein intake by increasing the fat intake further.

3 Always remember that Banting can only work if it reduces your calorie intake by making you less hungry. If Banting fails to reduce your hunger, allowing you to eat much less frequently – every six to twelve hours instead of every three hours as typically occurs in those following the Banting plan – then it will not produce the weight loss you require.

4 To this extent, obesity is a disease of the brain so that if the brain does not play along by reducing your hunger when you Bant, then you will not lose weight. In which case it may be necessary for you to either accept your weight or else to consciously reduce your calorie consumption by eating a calorie-restricted high-fat version of the LCHF. But, in general, consciously trying to reduce your calorie consumption is not a long-term solution.

RED, ORANGE AND GREEN: AN INTRODUCTION
THE LISTS TO LIVE YOUR LIFE BY

Green is eat-your-fill. You can go for broke without worrying about the carbohydrate content as all the foods on this list will be recommended for one of two reasons. The first will be because of their very low carb content – between 0–5 g carbohydrate per 100 g. The second reason would be because the volumes one would consume would not be likely to affect one's weight loss. The final reason an ingredient would land on this list will be because it has some other added health benefit.

We have tried to keep these lists as simple as possible. For more information on each ingredient, please see the lists on our website – realmealrevolution.com. Always obey your appetite. Although this is an 'eat-your-fill' list, we would encourage you to relearn what 'full' feels like.

It will be difficult to overdo your carbohydrate intake by sticking to this group of foods. Overeating protein is not recommended, so consume a moderate amount of animal protein at each meal. The aim is also to include as much fat as you are comfortable with. Fat won't harm you, and is pretty self-limiting, so feel free to enjoy as much of the healthy fats in this category as you wish, as often as you wish. The main purpose of fat while Banting is to reduce your appetite considerably. If you are feeling full, don't force it down!

Animal protein

(unless these have a rating, they are all 0 g/100 g)

All eggs

All meats, poultry and game

All natural and cured meats (pancetta, Parma ham, coppa, etc.)

All natural and cured sausages (salami, chorizo, etc.)

All offal (offal is highly recommended)

All seafood

Broths

Dairy

(please refer to realmealrevolution.com for important info on dairy)

Cottage cheese

Cream

Cream cheese

Full-cream Greek yoghurt

Full-cream milk

Hard cheeses

Soft cheeses

Fats

Any rendered animal fat

Avocado oil

Butter

Cheese – firm, natural, full-fat, aged cheeses (not processed)

Coconut oil

Duck fat

Ghee

Lard

Macadamia oil

Mayonnaise – full-fat (not made from seed oils)

Olive oil

Flavourings and condiments

All flavourings and condiments are OK, provided they do not contain sugars, preservatives or vegetable seed oils.

Nuts and seeds

Almonds

Flaxseeds (watch out for pre-ground flaxseeds; they quickly go rancid and become toxic)

Macadamia nuts

Pecans

Pine nuts

Pumpkin seeds

Sunflower seeds

Walnuts

Sweeteners

Erythritol granules

Stevia powder

Xylitol granules

Vegetables

All green, leafy vegetables (spinach, cabbage, lettuce, etc.)

Any other vegetables grown above the ground, except butternut squash

Artichoke hearts

Asparagus

Aubergines

Avocado

Broccoli

Brussels sprouts

Cabbage

Cauliflower

Celery

Courgettes

Leeks

Mushrooms

Olives

Onions

Peppers (all kinds)

Pumpkin

Radish

Spring onions

Tomatoes

Orange – Go slow and be aware. The Orange List contains foods which are 6–25 g carbohydrates per 100 g, to augment the foods from the Green List. Chart your carbohydrates without getting obsessive and still obtain an excellent outcome. If you want to lose weight fast, you will want to limit your carb intake as much as possible. For best results, try and keep your intake of carbs to less than 50 g (preferably less than 25 g) of net carbohydrates per day. Net carbohydrate is the total carbohydrates, minus the total fibre.

The quantities of each ingredient listed below are calculated to each contain a net carbohydrate count of 5 g. They are the RAW quantities.

This means that to reach your total carb-count for the day, you could (if aiming towards 25 g) have any five of these items in the quantity that has been mentioned. Please aim for less than 25 g. This is because your green listed ingredients will all contain a small amount of carbohydrate and you may well reach 40–50 g with a normal day of green listed foods.

Key

C	cup
D	dessertspoon
T	tablespoon
t	teaspoon
g	grams
ml	millilitres

Dairy and milks

Cottage cheese 2 C

Cream 12 T

Greek full-fat yoghurt 500 ml

Ricotta 3 C

Whole milk 2.2 C

Fruit

Apples ⅓ small apple, skin on

Apricot ⅓ C

Bananas ⅛ C mashed

Blackberries just under 1 C

Blueberries ⅓ C

Breadfruit ⅛ C

Cherries (sweet) ⅓ C

Clementines 1 large (75 g)

Figs ½ a large one

Gooseberries ½ C

Grapes (green) ⅕ C

Guavas ⅓ C chopped (or ½ a large one)

Jackfruit ⅛ C

Kiwi fruits ¼ C

Kumquats 2 fruits

Loquat ⅓ C

Lychees 2

Mangos, sliced, ⅕ C

Nectarines ½ C of sections

Oranges 1 very small or ⅓ C segments

Papaya ½ C cubes/slices

Passion fruit just under ⅛ C

Peaches ½ large

Pears ½ a C

Persimmon 1 small

Pineapple, sliced, ¼ C

Plums ⅓ C sliced

Pomegranate ¼ small

Prickly pears ½ C

Quinces 1

Raspberries 1 C

Rhubarb 1 C

Starfruit 1 C

Strawberries ½ C sliced

Tamarind pulp 1 T

Tangerine sections ¼ C

Watermelon ½ C sliced

Nuts

Cashews, raw, 1.5 D

Chestnuts, raw, 1 D

Hazelnuts just under a C

Pecans 1C

Pinenuts ½ C

Pistachio nuts ¼ C

Vegetables

Butternut squash ¼ C

Calabash 1 C

Carrots ½ a large one

Celeriac ½ C

Garlic ⅛ C

Ginger powder, just under 1 T

Green beans, 1 C

Hubbard squash ½ C

Jicama 1 C

Leeks ½ C

Okra 1 C

Onions ½ C

Palm hearts 1 T

Peas, green (fresh), just under ½ C

Plantain ⅛ C

Rutabagas just under 1 C

Shallots 2.5 T

Spaghetti squash just under 1 C

Spring onion, chopped, just under 1 C

Sweet potato ⅕ C

Taro ¼ C

Red contains the foods to avoid as they will be either toxic (i.e. seed oils, soya) or high-carbohydrate foods (i.e. potatoes, rice). We strongly suggest you avoid all the items on this list, or at best, eat them very occasionally and restrict the amount when you do. They will do nothing to help you in your attempt to reach your goal.

Baked goods/grain-based foods

All flours from grains – wheat flour, cornflour, rye flour, barley flour, rice flour, etc.

All forms of breads, buns, pancakes, muffins, tortillas and wheat products

All grains – wheat, oats, barley, rye, amaranth, quinoa, teff, etc.

Beans (dried)

Bran, mueslis, granolas and cereals

Breaded or battered foods

Buckwheat

Cakes, biscuits and confectionery

Corn products

Corn or maize products (polenta, popcorn, etc.)

Couscous

Crackers, cracker breads

Millet

Pasta and noodles

Rice products (rice, rice cakes, rice milk, etc.)

Sorghum

Spelt

Thickening agents such as gravy powder, maize starch or stock cubes

Beverages

Beer, cider

'Lite', 'zero' or diet drinks unless sweetened with xylitol, stevia or erythritol

Soft drinks of any description other than sparkling or still water

Dairy/dairy related

Cheese spreads, commercial dairy spreads

Coffee creamers

Commercial sweetened almond milk

Condensed milk

Ice cream

Puddings

Reduced-fat cow's milk

Rice milk

Soy milk

Fats

All seed oils (safflower, sunflower, canola, grapeseed, cottonseed, corn)

Chocolate (other than an occasional square of 70 per cent dark chocolate)

Commercial sauces, marinades and salad dressings

Hydrogenated or partially hydrogenated oils including margarines, vegetable oils, vegetable fats

Fruit and Vegetables

Fruit and vegetable juices of any kind (unless homemade with Green-Listed vegetables (page 41))

General

All fast food

All processed food

Any food with added sugar such as glucose, dextrose, etc.

Meat

All meats cured with excessive sugar

All unfermented soya (vegetarian 'protein')

Processed sausages and luncheon meats

Starchy vegetables

Beetroots

Legumes (dried – mange touts, green beans and other green fresh beans are fine)

Parsnips

Peanuts

Peas

Potatoes (regular)

Sweeteners

Agave nectar (or agave anything for that matter)

Artificial sweeteners (aspartame, acesulfame K, saccharin, sucralose, Splenda)

Cordials

Dried fruit

Fructose

Honey

Iced teas (sweetened)

Malt

Maple syrup

Sorbitol

Sugar

Sugared or commercially pickled foods with sugar

Sweets

Syrups of any kind

PRACTICAL ADVICE

Banting will change your life for the better and surprise you by how easy it is. Having said that, it helps to know exactly what you can expect.

To begin with, your first few days without carbs will be tough. You will have cravings and temptations and you are likely to have the odd slip-up. Don't be too hard on yourself if this is the case, but make sure it is the exception rather than the rule.

Right now, your body is addicted to carbs. But give it some time and willpower and you will soon be addicted to healthy foods and a healthy life.

The following practical advice has been compiled with the help of people who have recently done what you're about to do.

When you begin Banting you may wish to go immediately into ketosis (when your body burns fat for its fuel, instead of glucose). In this case you will want to limit yourself to around 30 to 50 grams of carbohydrate per day. It is essential to keep track of the carbs that you are consuming and it is easiest to do this by faithfully keeping a food diary, in which you record ALL the food that you eat during the course of each day, with the carb content of each item in a second column.

If you are carb-counting using a traditional carb counter, the column that you must pay attention to is NET CARBS. This is the total carb count minus the grams of fibre. Fibre, while a carbohydrate, is not absorbed into the body. Its function is to aid digestion, to keep one regular and to feed the flora present in the digestive tract.

You may experience some mildly unpleasant side effects for a few days while your body goes into ketosis, but ride the storm. Very soon you will feel more energetic and absolutely great as your insulin levels drop and your body gets used to burning fat for energy instead of glucose as it has been doing up to now.

Never allow yourself to go hungry. It doesn't matter if you eat a lot to begin with, as long as you eat the right food. Your appetite will soon diminish quite naturally and then you will truly be on the way.

Eat slowly, savouring each mouthful, and stop eating as soon as you feel full. Sip water while you eat. This will slow you down and make you feel full, having eaten less. In company, indulge in a lot of dinner-table chat. This will have the same effect.

Never eat standing up. Make it a rule always to sit at a table when you eat. It is dead easy to eat without even realizing it.

Ensure that you have a good breakfast every morning – a breakfast that contains enough fat and protein. Two eggs with a couple of slices of naturally cured bacon are easy and quick to prepare and make a very good start to the day – you will feel full for hours. In fact, the best test of your health might be for how long you do not need to eat after breakfast. If your breakfast is correct, you should not need to eat again until early afternoon.

Cut fruit out of your diet. You'll lose more weight by doing so. Instead, get your nutrients from vegetables. There is no benefit in fruit that you cannot find in vegetables.

When you are Banting, the bulk of your food intake will be in the form of Green-Listed vegetables. You need a wide variety of vegetables on a daily basis to provide the range of nutrients your body needs to function at its best.

Don't fret because you can't have toast under your egg. There are alternatives, delicious and Banting-friendly:

★ Cut off the ends of a large, ripe tomato and slice in half. Season and lightly fry in the bacon fat. Put your cooked eggs on top.

★ A couple of thick slices of seasoned aubergine, fried in butter and bacon fat, are equally delicious.

★ Or, add some butter to the bacon fat in the pan and lightly fry two large brown mushrooms. Use them instead of toast.

★ Eat at least two Banting seed crackers (see recipe on page 74) a day. This will keep you regular. Drink lots of water for the same reason and also to combat dehydration. The crackers can become soggy if exposed to air. If this happens, pop them into a warm oven for a short time and they will be restored to their former crispiness. Store them in a zipped plastic bag and they will stay fresh for ages.

★ Always have food with you. If you are not at home during the day, prepare a small lunchbox full of snacks to keep in your bag or briefcase – with some nuts, olives, seed crackers and/or Banting bread (see recipe on page 76), butter, sliced tomato, a couple of slices of cheese and/or meat, some dill pickles, slices of cucumber and bits of lettuce. You can make fabulous snacks with these ingredients. Don't forget salt and pepper. The salt is particularly important in the first week or two.

★ Make sure that there is a Banting soup or broth (see recipes on pages 64, 148, 180, 198 and 212) close at hand. If you have hunger pangs or feel deprived, a cup of heated soup will do wonders for your sense of well-being.

★ Spend time making your salads. The more varied the ingredients, the less boring they will be and the wider the range of nutrients they will contain.

★ Avocado is a must – very filling and sustaining because of its high oil content. It's also very delicious.

★ Blanch some green beans, asparagus and broccoli tips and keep them in the fridge to add to salads. Store some crumbled crispy bacon for the same purpose.

★ Have a little cream in your coffee and only a small quantity of full-cream milk in your tea. Remember that dairy products do have a relatively high carb content and you need to limit their intake. We suggest that you measure out a daily allowance of each and don't exceed it. The carb count of milk and cream must be faithfully factored into your daily carb allowance. Try to develop a taste for herbal and fruit teas that are taken without milk. Always use xylitol or one of the other permitted sweeteners (never the artificial kind) instead of sugar. (Always be aware that xylitol is highly toxic to dogs. Never feed them snacks prepared with xylitol).

★ Avoid sugar-free carbonated drinks. The artificial sweeteners that they contain are, quite simply, extremely bad for you.

★ Cook in butter and/or coconut oil, or lard. Olive oil is not suited to high-temperature cooking.

★ Remember the 'hand-minus-the-fingers' rule when it comes to your protein portion. Choose fatty cuts of meat as these will fill you up and keep you feeling full. Learn to recognize meat that is marbled with fat. This type of meat is best for a Banter. And never remove the skin from a piece of chicken or the fat from a lamb chop.

★ Have at least one hot meal a day. This will make you feel more 'normal' and satisfied. Include a variety of lightly steamed Green List vegetables, smothered in butter, in your hot meal. A couple of chunks of pumpkin, roasted in a mixture of melted butter and coconut oil, will make you feel extra-satisfied.

★ If you feel headachy, drink lots of water.

THE SPEED BUMP

In our experience some Banters kick off with great weight loss in the first few weeks but soon plateau and struggle to maintain momentum. We find this with Banters who typically have either a lot to lose, are extremely insulin resistant or have been overweight for a very long time. For these Banters we developed an extra set of rules to clarify a few grey areas. If you find yourself stuck in a weight-shedding plateau, pay extra-special attention to the following commandments.

THE TEN COMMANDMENTS OF BEGINNER BANTING

1   Eat enough fat. This is central to Banting – animal fat does not make you fat – you need to eat it. Small amounts (your body will tell you how much) make you feel full, which stops you from overeating. It also gives you long-lasting energy so in time you won't have that carb craving.

2   Eat enough vegetables. This is high fat, not high protein. Don't forget to eat your greens with every meal.

3   Don't snack. Initially, while you're in carb-cold-turkey you will crave everything and will most likely need to snack to keep your sanity. Once you've come off carbs, the only reason you should feel the need to snack is if you are not eating a fatty enough meal or a large enough breakfast. Eventually, snacking and Banting become like oil and water.

4   Don't lie to yourself. Eating carbs that are perceived to be proteins like legumes, peanuts and quinoa can be detrimental. Pay special attention to the Red List on pages 44–45. A red-listed item is either toxic or will make you fat and should be avoided at all costs.

5   Don't over- or under-eat. New Banters get nervous about the idea of not snacking and end up stuffing themselves completely. Fear not, with a high-enough volume of fat in each meal, a reasonable portion of food should carry you to your next meal time. Even though the theory is that if you eat enough fat you should stay fuller for longer, you should still be careful that you're not forcing down food. Get used to the portion size you need to keep you full and try to stick to one serving. Eat slowly, drink water and only eat until full; not starving nor stuffed, just full. Get used to eating more substantial, less frequent meals. One serving per meal, one meal at a time!

6   Don't eat too much protein. We can't stress this enough. This is not high-protein eating. You really don't need more than 80 to 90 g of meat or fish with any meal. The main aim is reducing carbs, then increasing fat. Protein stays the same or could even decrease.

7   Be alert. You could be eating secret carbs in supposed healthy products or pre-made meals. Check the packaging on everything you eat. Anything containing more than 5 per cent carbs should be avoided at all costs. Remember: that diet milkshake you always buy may be low in fat (which is pointless) but it will be loaded with sugar. When you start looking at product labels you'll realize why it's so hard to lose weight. Almost everything has sugar in it! In *The Real Meal Revolution*, we keep it even more simple – if it even has a label, perhaps avoid it anyway.

8   Avoid too many fruits and nuts. Remember firstly that fruit is laced with fructose, which is perceived as 'good sugar'. Sugar is sugar and regardless of its perceived 'goodness', it needs to be controlled. Of course refined sugar is a lot more poisonous so while natural sugars are less likely to kill you, they will do nothing for weight loss. Berries are safe but should be restricted (refer to the Orange List on page 43) and nuts, while low in carbs, should be restricted too – only a handful as a snack if you absolutely have to. Remember that roasted nuts are not good; raw nuts are great.

9   Control your dairy. Although dairy is good for you, it does contain carbs and can be a stumbling block for some. In your Banting beginning, perhaps avoid eating too much dairy. Butter is still good. Dairy is actually way too complex to explain in this paragraph. Many people shed weight while eating heaps of dairy, while others don't even budge. There are numerous reasons for this. Please visit realmealrevolution.com for more information on dairy.

10   Be strong!

THE ELEVENTH COMMANDMENT!

Watch what you drink. We're faced with a dilemma here. We're trying to promote health and overall well-being so promoting booze is not in our interest as alcohol is highly toxic. Dry wines, most spirits, low-energy beers and a few other drinks are safe BUT that is only from a carb perspective. Alcopops, normal beer, any spirit mixer or cocktail will halt any weight loss you're experiencing. It's easy for us to promote low-carb alcoholic beverages but one needs to remember that a low-carb 5 per cent vol. beer is still 5 per cent toxic.

Alcohol is also really good at draining motivation, lowering inhibitions, impairing driving ability, and, and, and …!

So we, the authors, leave drinking to you. Consider the Eleventh Commandment our 'drinking disclaimer'. You're a grown-up and how much booze you choose to consume is up to you.

A COUPLE OF NOTES ...

If you are not getting the results you would like, considering having a blood test for thyroid imbalance, such as TSH, T4, T3 and antibodies. Find a qualified health professional or knowledgeable integrative GP who knows how to read these imbalances according to the most recent guidelines, and what to do about them. In the case of women having fertility treatment, being on the Pill or going through menopause, these all contribute and need to be tweaked for the person concerned – they can potentially play a role in weight-loss prevention.

And consider this: stress releases too much cortisol and builds a spare tyre around even a slim waist. So not only can stress lead to you flipping out mentally, but it trips you up physically too.

This is not *The Real Meal Revolution* for nothing. Losing weight is one thing but staying healthy is something completely different. We want you to eat REAL food. Do your best to stay away from processed junk, regardless of the carb content. It might help you lose weight, but who knows what else it does to your body. A rule of thumb would be, if you can tell what food it is without looking at the package, the chances are that it's real. For example: a chicken nugget does not look like chicken and should be avoided. Chicken breasts look like chicken breasts and should be enjoyed!

THE KEY POINTS OF BANTING

★ Eat REAL meat or products made with real meat and no fillers. Processed luncheon meats and tinned meats are a no-no. Organic and pasture-fed meats make the best choice.

★ All fish and seafood is great.

★ Fresh vegetables grown above the ground are generally perfect. But remember, no peas or butternut squash! (Pumpkin is a delicious Green-Listed alternative to the latter.)

★ Most vegetables grown in the soil are out – carrots, potatoes, beetroot, turnips and parsnips. Onions are fine in moderation and spring onions are good. An occasional sweet potato is OK (just!) but must be stringently factored into your daily carb allocation.

★ Pulses are out – legumes, dried beans, split peas (also peanuts, which are actually legumes and not nuts).

★ Grains, as you know by now, are a big NO – wheat, corn, barley, rye, spelt, oats, buckwheat, etc.

★ All fruit is out for the next six weeks. Thereafter, a few berries now and then may be OK, depending on your level of insulin resistance.

★ Eggs are great – really good for you. Eat as many as you like.

★ Certain nuts are fine but these must be eaten in moderation because they do contain carbs. Almonds are good, as are macadamias, Brazil nuts, hazelnuts, pecans, walnuts and pine nuts (no cashews, pistachios, chestnuts or peanuts). It is preferable to buy raw nuts and roast them yourself.

★ Seeds are good – pumpkin, sesame, flax and sunflower. Don't buy pre-ground flaxseed as ground flaxseed oxidizes (or rusts) very quickly and oxidized material, especially oils, is very damaging to the body. Always grind flaxseed immediately before you use it.

★ Yes to healthy oils – olive, walnut, macadamia, avocado and coconut. Of these, only coconut oil is suitable for cooking. The rest can be added to cooked food for extra flavour.

★ NO seed or grain oils of any kind are allowed.

★ Avoid most ready-made sauces and marinades. They are usually packed with the bad stuff. Make your own – dead easy if you have a blender or food processor and equally delicious.

★ Moderate quantities of dairy products are allowed. You may have to cut down your dairy intake, or even cut them out completely, if you are struggling to lose weight or if you are diabetic.

★ NO SUGAR in any shape or form! Check ingredients on labels.

★ No processed foods.

★ Salt is fine.

★ It is best to cut alcohol from your diet while you are trying to lose weight. Alcohol will definitely sabotage your best efforts. But if this is unworkable for you, drink alcohol in moderation and remember to factor the carb content into your daily allowance too.

NOW FOR THE GOOD STUFF

As chefs, we are programmed to frown upon products like pre-packed pastes, marinades, ready-made stocks, sauces and artificial sweeteners. The truth is, for a lot of people, life is too short to find and mince half a cup of young organic green-stem Peruvian garlic.

That being said, the recipes in this book have been written to suit the parameters set out by the Prof and Sally-Ann. If you can't find an ingredient or you don't feel like crushing, mincing or fermenting, feel free to add in something else or a pre-made product you feel comfortable using (we frown upon the non-organic, nasty plastic bottle kind). We can only encourage you to, wherever possible, go for the option that is the most real. We want you to eat real food!

Once you have nailed the basics, we encourage you to veer off the beaten track a little. Mix it up. Try and modify the recipes, make notes and have fun, that's what we did.

Eating like this will involve a mind shift. Sadly, a toasted cheese sandwich will no longer be a regular snack (unless you use our carb-free bread on page 76). You'll have to start eating burgers with a knife and fork and, finally, you'll find breakfast to be a slightly bigger mission than pouring milk over some deathly and delicious chocolate puffed rice.

You might also find yourself spending more than usual on food in the beginning but if you stick to your guns and follow our guidelines, your appetite will subside and you'll learn a few tricks for saving money. Just take the hit for the first week or two – you'll notice a huge change once you get over the 'cold turkey' stage.

We have tried to build a collection of recipes that are practical, accessible and that will fit in with your everyday life. A lot of the recipes are probably part of your life already and you just didn't realize they were Banting. Those are the ones we obviously found easier to develop.

The key to giving up any element of your diet is to use the next best thing to emulate it. We've put in some practical substitutes for mashed potato, rice and a good alternative noodle recipe. There is even a recipe in here for fake lasagne sheets.

Everyone has varying levels of insulin resistance so the rules may not need to be as strict for you. For safety's sake, the recipes in this book are almost certainly Green Listed unless otherwise noted. There is no need to start carb counting; they're all safe.

Remember, when reading these recipes, to keep in the back of your head that when we say 'meat', we mean pasture-fed, when we say 'vegetable', we mean organic, when we say 'oil', we mean extra-virgin cold pressed and finally, we *never* say 'starch'!

REMEMBER: REAL FOOD IS GOOD FOOD. AS YOU BEGIN THIS ADVENTURE, WE ENCOURAGE YOU TO TRY AS MANY OF THE DELICIOUS, SPECIALLY-DEVELOPED BANTING RECIPES AS POSSIBLE.

★ ★ ★ ★ ★

YOU WILL SOON DISCOVER HOW MUCH YOU CAN ENJOY GOOD FOOD WHILE LOSING WEIGHT AND GETTING HEALTHY.

THE BANTING TOOLKIT

Before you start with the exciting stuff, there are some basics here that will make your transition into Banting a seamless process.

The things you will miss the most like mashed potato, rice, breads, rubbish mass-produced mayo and energy drinks are all replaced here with good healthy substitutes. Our advice is to get to grips with these basics as soon as possible. Having them stocked in the fridge or freezer will make sticking to your game plan a hundred times easier.

The basic recipes in this section will help enormously when you first start out on your Banting journey. They're all packed with flavour and provide fantastic fats and low-carb alternatives to some of your favourite toxic foods.

Finding and harvesting fats

How to render fat of any kind

Hot chocolate fat shake

Bullet coffee

A Basic broth

Banting mayonnaise

Mashed cauliflower or 'cauli-mash'

Cauliflower rice or 'cauli-rice'

Courgette noodles or 'courgetti'

Nutty crackers

Banting bread

Carb-free pasta

Coconut crêpes

Carb-free tortillas or cauli-wraps

Spicy bacon nuts

Roasted courgette hummus

Hot smoked fish pâté

Fermented pickles

FINDING AND HARVESTING FATS

When you starting eating like this, the first thing you'll have to get your head around eating is fat. Everyone has a problem eating fat when they change their diet. The fat is good. You won't die. You need it. You can now shamelessly eat the fat off a lamb chop and that delicious crispy chicken skin. Rendered animal fat is one of the best things to cook with. It is stable at high temperatures and very good for the heart too. We mean it!

Some cuts of meat are up to 40 per cent fat. If you cut the fat off, which you have paid for, you are literally throwing money away. You are also throwing perfectly good and necessary food away. Another huge incentive to collect animal fat is the fact that coconut and extra virgin olive oil cost an arm and a leg. Apart from the dressings, you can swap rendered animal fat for oil in almost every recipe. Using rendered animal fat could literally save you a fortune.

HOW TO RENDER FAT OF ANY KIND

1   Place whatever fat you have accumulated from cleaning your meat or poultry in an oven tray and leave it in the oven at 120–140°C (Gas ½–1) for up to an hour or so.

2   You will know the chunks of fat have finished rendering because they will be crispy right the way through. Simply pour the fat out of the tray into a jar, leave to cool and store in the fridge until needed.

Often when we take on eating a little more fat than usual, we tend to feel slightly overwhelmed and food seems over-rich. Although we do eventually get used it, it is possible to soothe the richness by drinking hot, refreshing drinks. Hot water with lemon slices, ginger and mint is a popular favourite as well as any tea infusions. Avoid powdered shakes and the like.

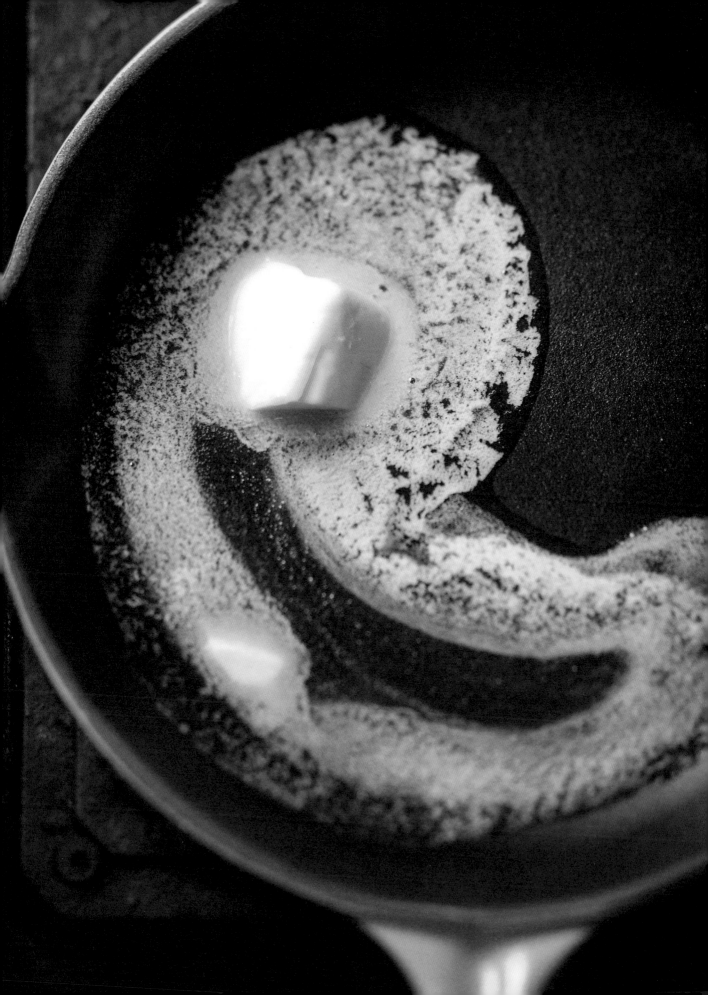

HOT CHOCOLATE FAT SHAKE

MAKES 1

How to use these drinks: Fat is used as an appetite suppressant. If you're full after a meal and stay feeling full for hours afterwards, you will not need a fat shake. This is for those who simply cannot control their appetites or for those who wish to eat less. Don't force it down. For that matter, don't force anything down. If you can't finish it all at once, leave it aside and sip it throughout the day. Always eat until you're satisfied. If you can't get satisfied, get a fat shake.

150 ml full cream milk

50 g butter (unsalted, if possible)

50 ml coconut oil

200 ml coconut cream

1 tbsp cocoa powder or sugar-free hot chocolate

¼ tsp salt

★ You can have this hot or cold. For the hot version, warm all of the ingredients in a small saucepan, then blitz with a stick blender. For the cold one, simply blitz and enjoy (you may need to melt the butter and coconut oil in a small saucepan first).

Note: Using the above base, you can add any flavouring you like. Fresh or frozen berries, vanilla extract or even some almond or macadamia nut butter are all good flavourings. Also, feel free to add a touch of xylitol or few drops of stevia for sweetness.

BULLET COFFEE

SERVES 1

1 cup coffee (filter coffee or a standard Americano)

2 tbsp butter

2 tbsp coconut oil

★ While the coffee is still as steaming hot as possible, mix all of the ingredients together and process either in a food processor or in a jug while blending with a stick blender.

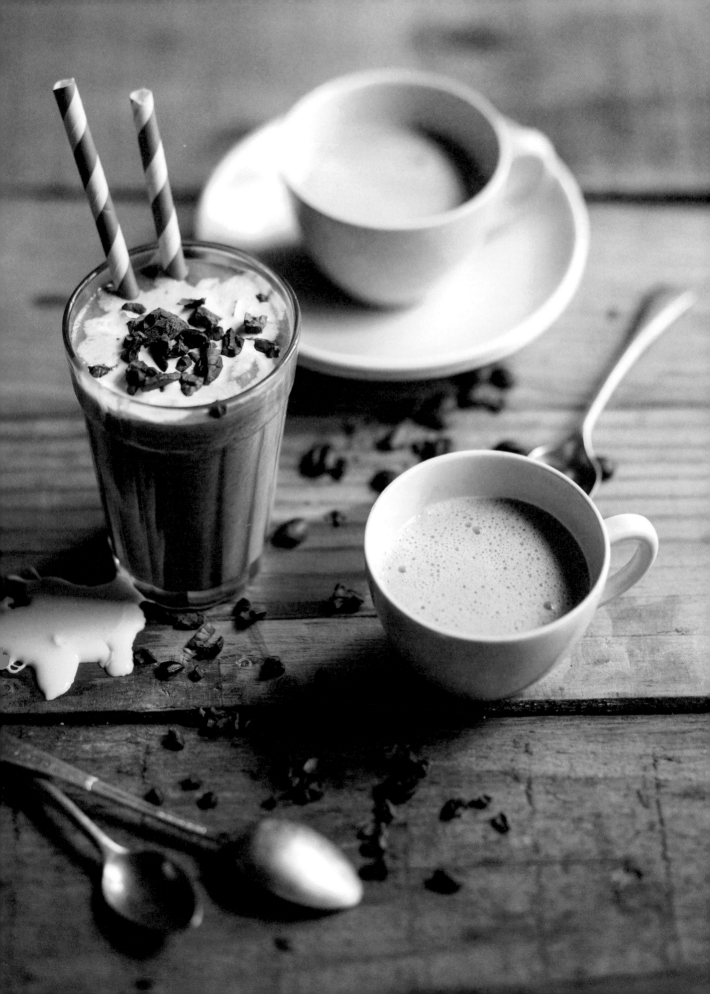

A BASIC BROTH

Bone broths are highly nutritious. When Banting kicks off some may experience muscle cramps or an uncomfortable bowel. This bone broth is the best tonic for such temporary ailments. Hint: it is 100 per cent normal for a layer of scum and fat to collect on the surface of your stock or broth. The rule of thumb here is if the fat or scum is murky it should be skimmed off the top and thrown out. If it is clear and golden it should be kept. You can either scoop it off the top and use for sautéing at a later stage or simply drink it with the broth as it is.

500 g bones of any kind

1 carrot cut into thumb-sized chunks

½ onion

1 stick of celery cut into chunks

2 large leeks cut into chunks

1 bay leaf

5 peppercorns

★ If the bones are not already roasted, roast them in the oven at 190°C (Gas 5) until they are lightly browned (approx. 45 minutes– 1 hour). You can use them raw; We personally like the roasted flavour it gives to the broth.

★ Place all the ingredients, as is, into a medium-sized pot and cover with water.

★ Place on the lowest heat and let it simmer away for up to 12 hours. Avoid letting the broth get to a rolling boil; it makes it go murky, which in turn makes it look unappetizing but more importantly it gives it a slightly slimy mouthfeel.

★ Taste the broth – it should taste strongly of the bones it came from (you should taste beef if you used beef bones). Once it has taken on this flavour, strain through a sieve and freeze for 3 months or use it straight away.

Note: The bone-simmering part is the most important. The above flavourings can be added at a later stage if you don't have them to hand. Also, each protein has certain complimentary herbs and spices which we encourage you to play with. Fish broth does well with lemon and white wine, beef works well with rosemary and chicken is good with thyme. Be creative!

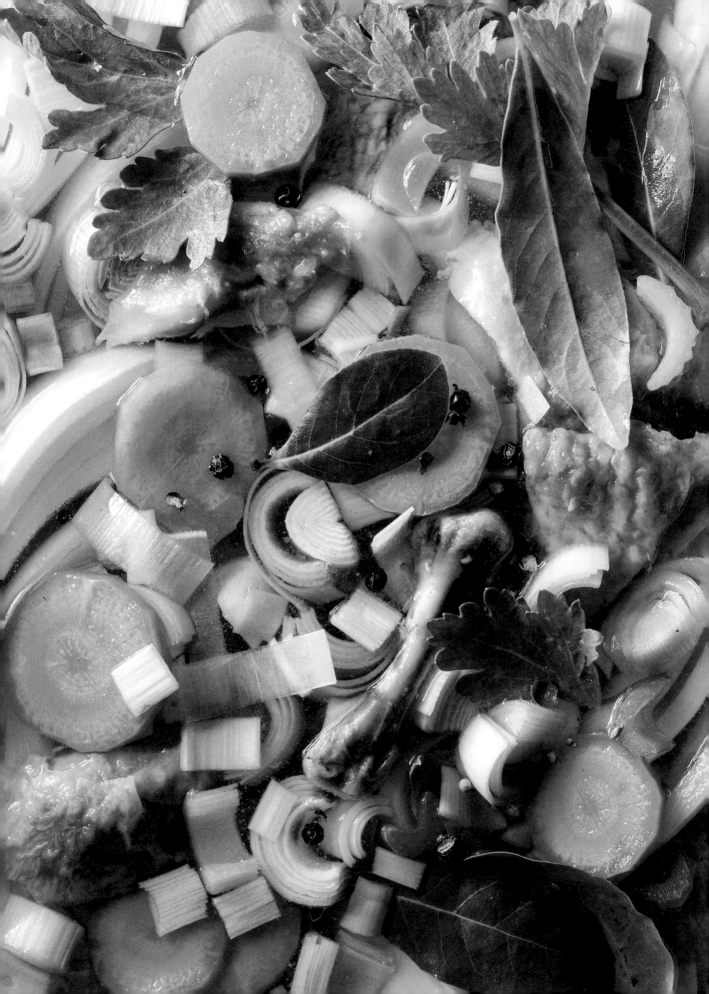

BANTING MAYONNAISE

MAKES 350 ML

Almost all of the mayonnaise you can buy in the shops is made with vegetable oils, which are Banting blasphemy. We recommend you stay away from all of them and make your own safe and delicious mayo. You can add anything to it just like a normal mayo, so go wild with flavour combinations.

2 egg yolks
1 tbsp Dijon mustard
Juice of 1 lemon
¾ cup coconut oil, extra-virgin
¾ cup quality olive oil
Salt and pepper

★ Combine the egg yolks, mustard and lemon juice in a food processor.

★ Melt the coconut oil in a small pot until it turns to liquid (or place the container in a bowl of boiling water). Avoid heating it too much or it will curdle the eggs.

★ While the food processor turns on a fast speed, slowly pour the coconut oil and the olive oil into the egg mixture.

★ Season to taste. This should keep for up to two weeks in the fridge in an airtight container.

Note: If you bulk this up with thick unsweetened Greek yoghurt you can make it go a lot further. Coconut oil is outrageously expensive so it needs to be stretched as far as possible. The yoghurt also tames the coconut flavour, which can be little too strong for some people.

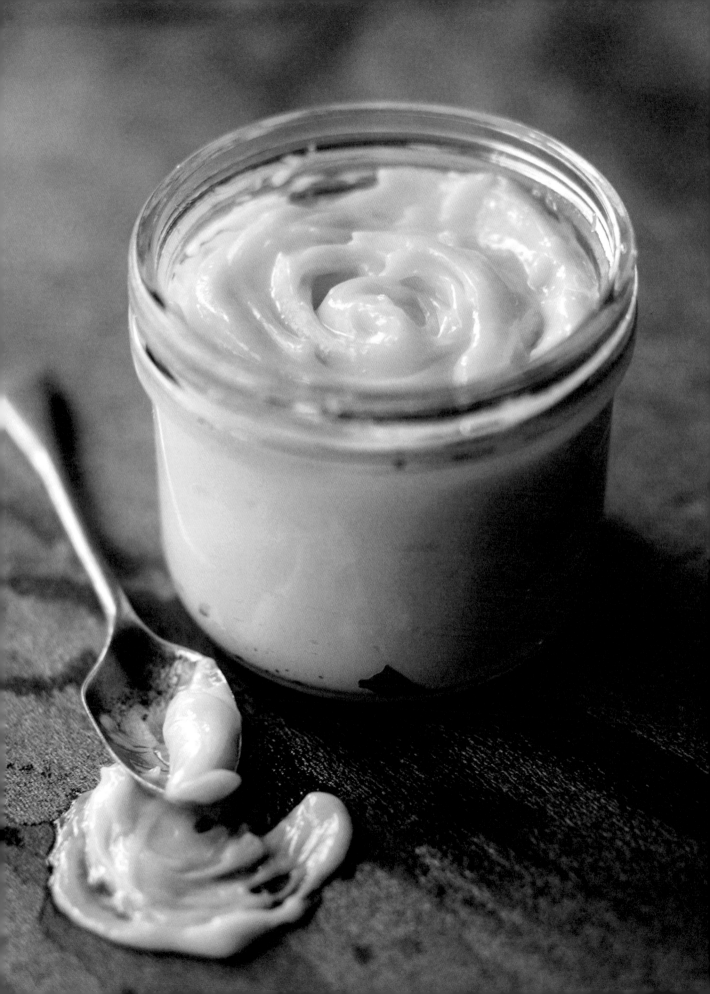

MASHED CAULIFLOWER OR 'CAULI-MASH'

SERVES 4

When this book launched in South Africa, the price of cauliflower saw a 400 per cent increase because everyone went cauliflower mad. This is because cauli-mash is one of the fundamentals of Banting. By cheating the eyes you cheat the mind, and this starts with lying to your eyes about mashed potatoes. In restaurants, cauliflower mash is often served as a 'fancy' substitute to standard-issue mash, but this should become one of your everyday staples.

800 g cauliflower, broken into florets

80 g butter

Salt and pepper

★ Steam the cauliflower until it is soft (always steam and never boil your vegetables; boiling will literally wash the nutrients away).

★ Using a stick blender or a food processor, purée the cauliflower until it is smooth.

★ While continuing to purée, add the butter and beat until smooth and silky.

★ Season to taste and serve.

Note: Just like mashed potatoes, you can flavour cauli-mash with absolutely anything. It is brilliant with roast garlic and thyme.

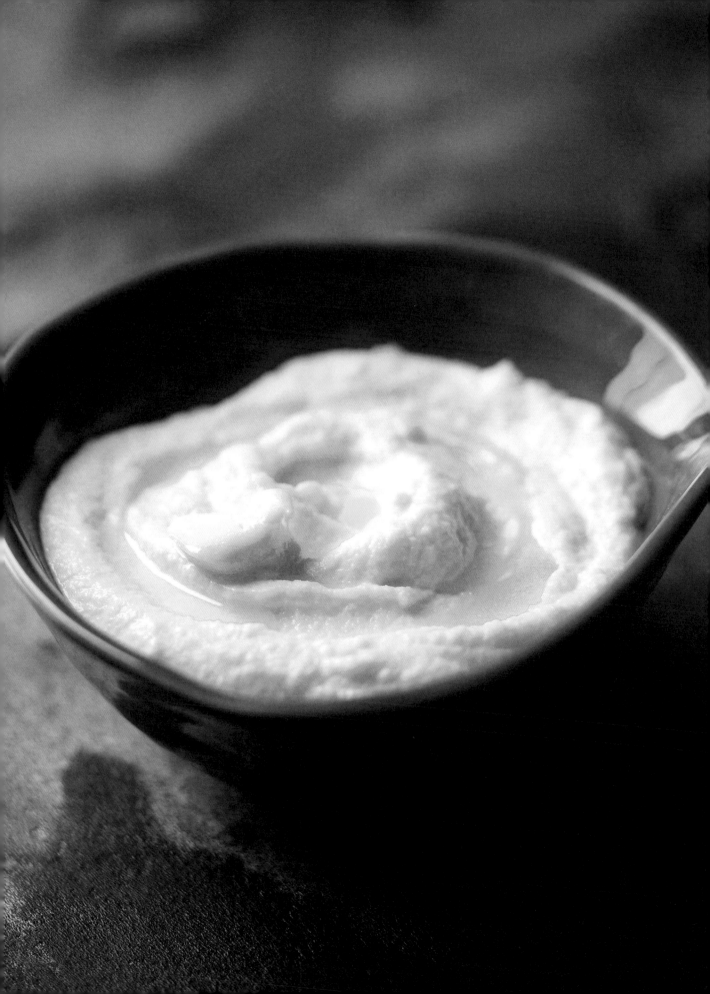

CAULIFLOWER RICE OR 'CAULI-RICE'

SERVES 4

Just like mashed potato, rice is one of those side dishes that very few people are able to go without. Cauli-rice is a 'non-grain grain' so you can eat as much as you like with no shame!

800 g cauliflower (cut or broken into florets)

100 g butter or coconut oil

1 onion

★ In a food processor, pulse the raw cauliflower until you reach a 'couscous' consistency.

★ Melt the butter or coconut oil in a heavy-based frying pan and sauté the onions until soft.

★ Add the cauliflower and mix through the onions and butter.

★ Leave the heat on low to medium and place the lid on top of the pot. Allow the cauli-rice to cook for 5–8 minutes and either set aside or serve immediately.

Note: You can add just about anything to cauli-rice. You will need to adjust the water content if you are adding it to a standard recipe to replace rice as the cauli-rice requires no water to cook. It also doesn't hold its texture very well over long cooking periods, so things like paella or risotto will need the cauli-rice added at the end of the cooking time rather than at the beginning.

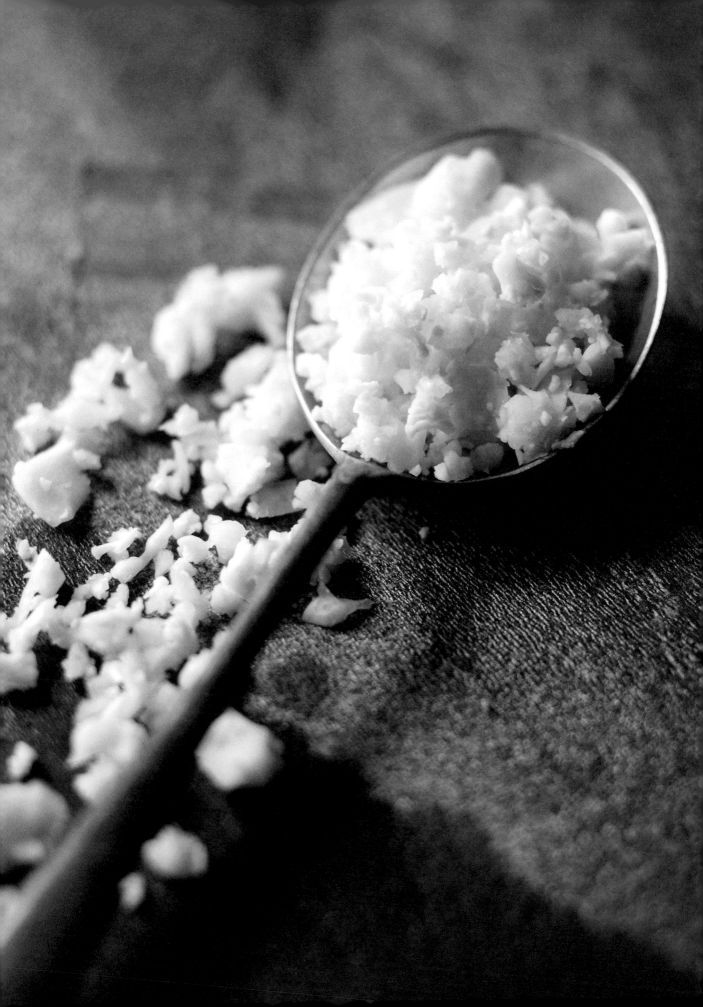

COURGETTE NOODLES OR 'COURGETTI'

SERVES 2

Courgette noodles are the best option for Banting pasta. They hold their shape nicely and they have great flavour. The other thing I like about courgettes is that they go well with almost every flavour profile. You can serve them with literally anything.

400 g large courgettes
(the bigger they are, the
easier they are to slice)

1 tbsp coconut oil

★ Slice the courgettes into long julienne strips using either a knife, a mandolin, a shredder/peeler or a Chinese slicer. They should resemble noodles.

★ Heat a frying pan on a high heat and add the coconut oil.

★ Throw in the courgettes and sauté them, stirring constantly.

★ Sauté for a few minutes until they are just cooked, then remove from the heat and add them to whatever sauce or recipe you like.

Note: You could use these noodles as a substitute for pasta with any pasta sauce, in an Asian broth or a stir-fry, or just on their own as a light side dish with some grilled chicken or fish.

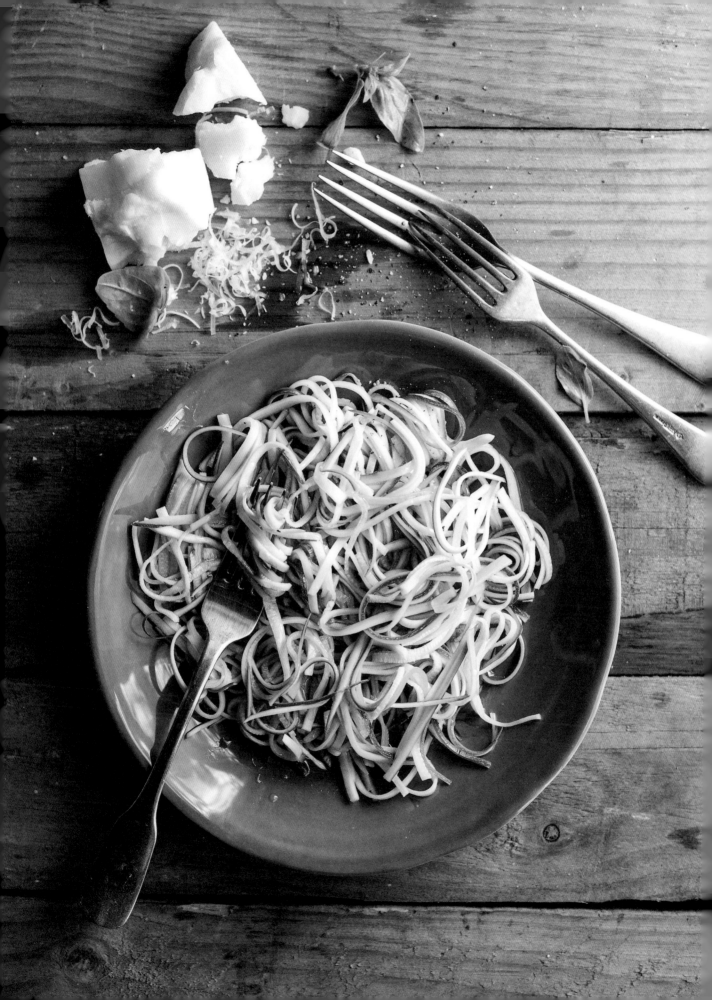

NUTTY CRACKERS

Seed crackers are the perfect alternative to your standard bread crackers. There are some more unusual ingredients here but don't worry; you can get them from any health food shop. The crackers also keep very well in a sealed container.

100 g sunflower seeds

100 g pumpkin seeds

60 g flaxseeds

100 g sesame seeds

3 tbsp psyllium husks

400 ml water

1 tsp salt

★ Preheat your oven to 150°C (Gas 2). If you have a fan oven, make sure the fan is on.

★ In a mixing bowl, combine all of the ingredients and leave the mixture to stand until it is thick and pliable, about 10 or 15 minutes.

★ Spread the mixture out as thinly as possible on a baking tray lined with a silicone mat or baking parchment (silicone paper). You may need two trays. The mix should have no holes in it.

★ Bake the trays for an hour, checking them every 15 minutes. You may need to rotate them away from the hot spots in the oven.

★ They usually take about 1 hour 20 minutes to cook. Once they are lightly browned and crisp, remove from the oven and leave to cool.

★ Once cooled, break them into any size you like and store in an airtight container.

Note: These go perfectly with any natural, non-processed or homemade pâtés or dips. A personal favourite would be a nutty cracker with a thick layer of liver pâté and some charcuterie. DO IT!

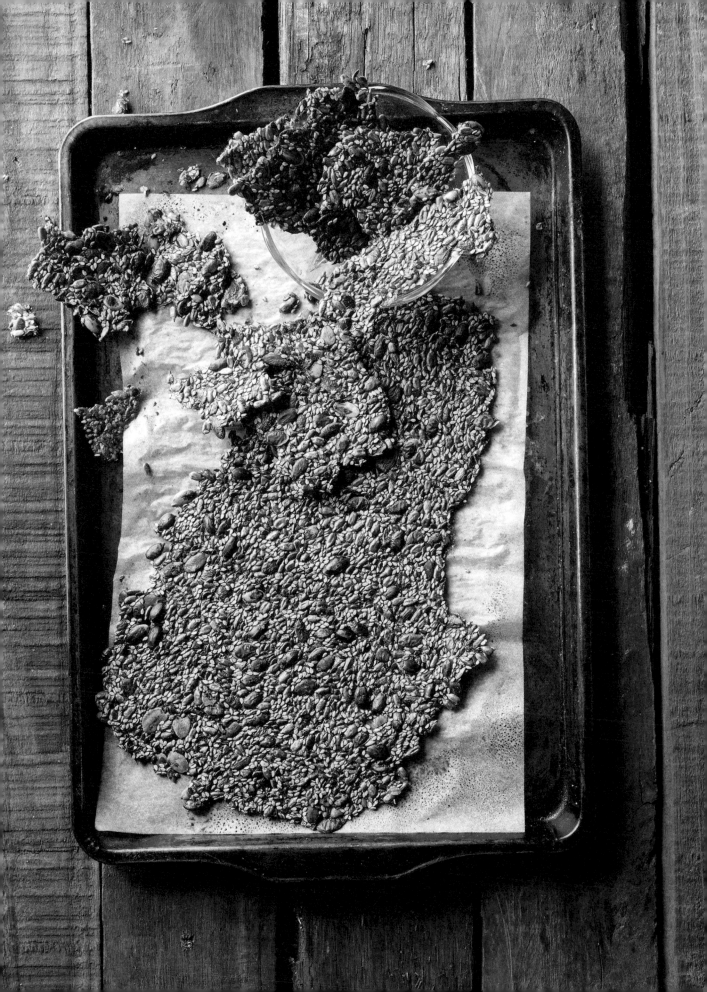

BANTING BREAD

MAKES 1 SMALL LOAF

Bread is by far hardest thing in life to go without when you first change the way you eat. It's also near-impossible to find zero-carb bread that genuinely does have zero carbs, let alone one that tastes good. This recipe ticks all of those boxes as well as being 'toastable', which is an added bonus. You may now eat cheese toasties again!

Just a note on flax seed: please buy the seeds whole and grind them in a coffee grinder. The recipe will not work if you buy the pre-ground flax. Pre-ground flax contains none of the oils found in home-ground flax as it is a by-product of the oil extraction process. You may not be familiar with xanthan gum, but it can be easily found in health food shops or in the baking section of larger supermarkets.

2 whole eggs

½ cup water

5 tbsp olive oil

250 g golden flax seeds, ground

1 tsp baking powder

1 tsp salt

1 tsp xylitol

½ tsp xanthan gum

2 tsp sesame seeds

25 g whole brown flax seeds

1 tsp fennel seeds, bashed a bit in a pestle and mortar

40 g pumpkin seeds

5 egg whites, whisked to stiff peaks

★ Preheat the oven to 180°C (Gas 4) and grease a small loaf tin (approx. 150 x 100 x 75 mm).

★ In a small bowl, whisk together the whole eggs and the water with the olive oil.

★ In a large bowl mix the dry ingredients together.

★ Add the wet ingredients to the dry ingredients and mix until combined.

★ Fold in the egg whites until completely incorporated.

★ Pour the mixture into the loaf tin and bake for 45 minutes.

★ Cool and serve. This bread can be kept for a few days and is perfect for freezing, sealed in an airtight bag, for up to 2 months.

Note: This is a basic seed loaf – check out realmealrevolution. com for some other awesome bread recipes. You could always add in extra bits and bobs for a little excitement. Try adding some cheese into the mix or chopped sundried tomatoes. The possibilities are endless.

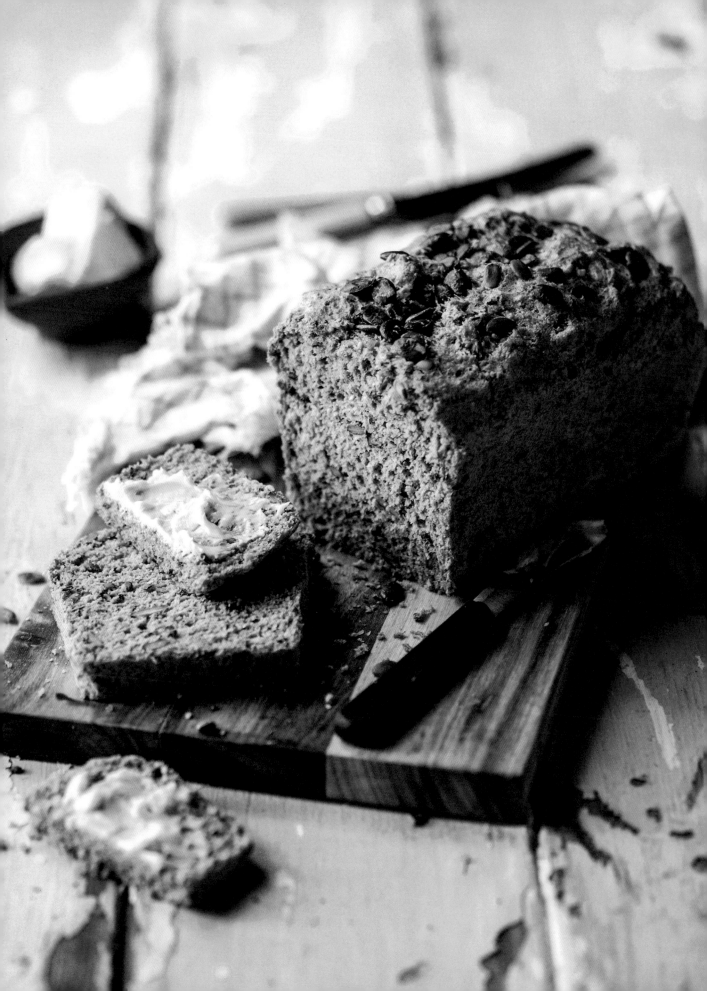

CARB-FREE PASTA

Pop on to realmealrevolution.com/realmeal-tv for a quick video on how to get this pasta perfect every time.

4 eggs
125 g cream cheese
½ cup psyllium husks
Coconut flour for dusting

★ In a food processor, blend all of the ingredients until smooth, then leave the mixture to thicken for between 10 and 15 minutes.

★ Using coconut flour for dusting, roll the pasta into sheets and set aside.

★ Cook this pasta in the same way as normal pasta but for a much shorter period. These should only take between 30 and 60 seconds.

★ You can refresh them in cold water or eat them immediately, but don't leave them in the water for too long or they will go soggy very quickly. Best to eat them fresh and steaming out of the pot.

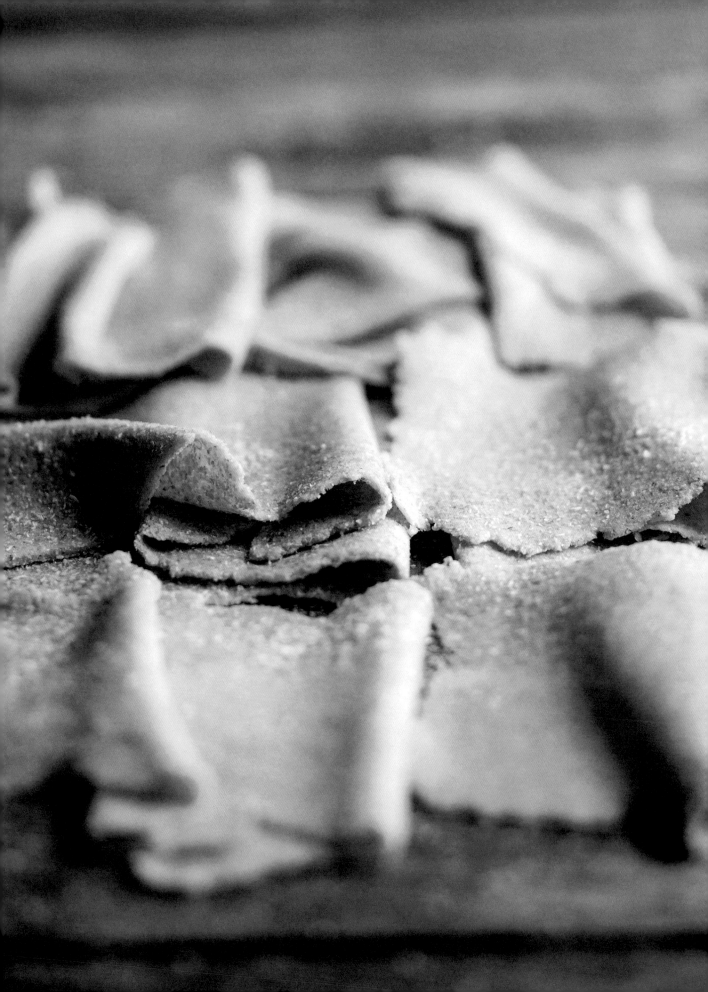

COCONUT CRÊPES

MAKES 4 PANCAKES

Another cracking recipe for your Banting arsenal! These are brilliant with fresh fruit, berries and cream or savoury with anything from crispy duck to quesadillas.

4 tbsp coconut flour
2 tsp psyllium husks
¼ tsp baking powder
8 egg whites
8 tbsp coconut milk
pinch of salt
Butter for frying

★ Using a stick blender or a food processor, blend all of the ingredients together.

★ Leave the batter to sit for about ten minutes, so the psyllium can expand and bind the batter.

★ Then melt some butter in a large frying pan and cook each pancake on a low temperature. Remember, these are not wheat pancakes so the batter will not be as robust as usual. Handle them gently until they are cooked.

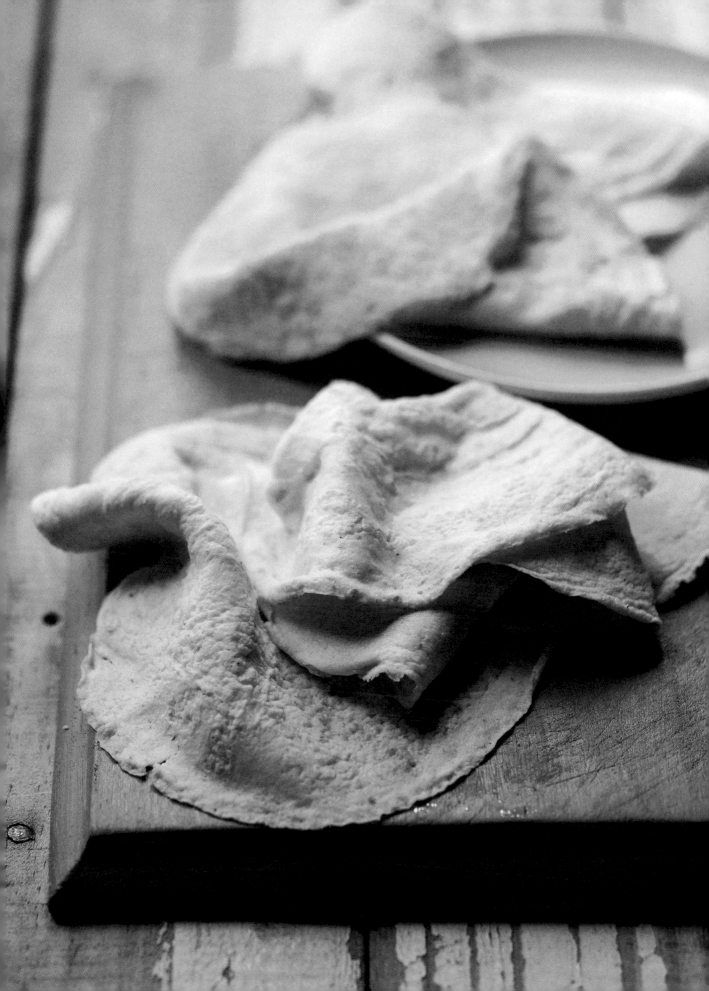

CARB-FREE TORTILLAS OR CAULI-WRAPS

MAKES 6

Cauli-wraps are another superb 'fake carb' for which we owe thanks to the cauliflower. They won't keep as long as a standard tortilla so you'll want to freeze them and defrost as needed. These guys can get a bit tricky so if you're not 100 per cent confident, check out realmealrevolution.com/realmeal-tv for a quick video showing you how to get these tortillas perfect every time.

Before you start – you **must** read these extra tips:

This dough is not normal dough as it contains zero gluten. You need to be very gentle when rolling it out, as gluten is the stuff that holds dough together and makes it stretchy. Smaller, gentler rolling actions are less likely to damage the dough while you roll it out. Lifting the dough, turning it and dusting it regularly will increase your odds of a perfect tortilla. You will need a liberal dusting of flour as this is not a normal dough that will get tougher the more it is worked. Coconut flour is better than almond flour (ground almonds); plus, almond flour is ridiculously expensive. Add the psyllium to the mix while it is as hot as possible to guarantee optimal absorption.

800 g cauliflower, cut into florets

6 tbsp psyllium husks

2 eggs

¼ tsp salt

Coconut flour for dusting

★ Steam the cauliflower until it is very soft.

★ Drain off all excess moisture and then purée the florets in a food processor or using a stick blender.

★ Now, add the psyllium husks, eggs and salt and blend the mixture again. It is vitally important to use a blender for this as it guarantees the maximum effect of the psyllium husk, which is the gluten-like binding agent.

★ Leave it to stand for about 15 minutes to thicken into a pliable dough.

★ Break the mixture into six balls and roll each ball out into a tortilla shape. Try and get them as thin as possible, dusting with coconut flour as often as needed.

★ In a large, heavy-based frying pan, dry fry each tortilla on a medium heat until they are nicely coloured on the outside and cooked on the inside.

Note: For the same, if not better results, you could substitute butternut or sweet potato for cauliflower. Just be aware that the carb content shoots up a fair amount.

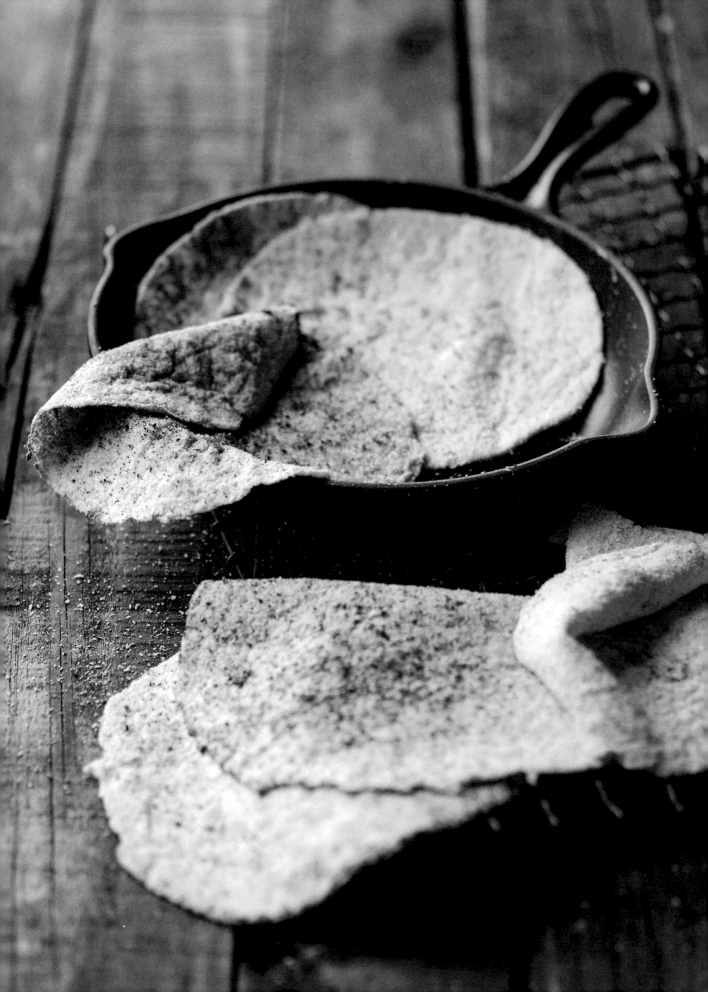

SPICY BACON NUTS

MAKES 800 G

Plain mixed nuts actually make one of the best Banting snacks. This is just taking it to the next level.

250 g streaky bacon rashers

4 cups assorted nuts (almonds, hazelnuts, pecan, Brazil, macadamia and cashew nuts)

2 tsp unsalted butter

½ tsp ground cumin

½ tsp cayenne pepper

½ tsp ground cinnamon

1 big pinch freshly ground nutmeg

1 tsp salt

★ Grill the bacon in a greased oven tray until crispy.

★ Remove from the fat and cut the rashers into small lardons. Reserve the fat for the next step.

★ Toast the nuts in a large, heavy-based dry pan until they go golden.

★ Add the bacon fat and butter and cook until the nuts begin to darken.

★ Add the spices and fry them in the butter until they become fragrant.

★ Now add a few drops of water and the bacon and toss everything together.

★ Tip the nuts back onto an oven tray lined with paper towel and pop them back in the oven for another 5 minutes at 160°C (Gas 3) to dry out properly. Salt, cool and store in an airtight container.

Note: If you keep a permanent supply of these in the cupboard, you could also use them to add some extra interest to salads.

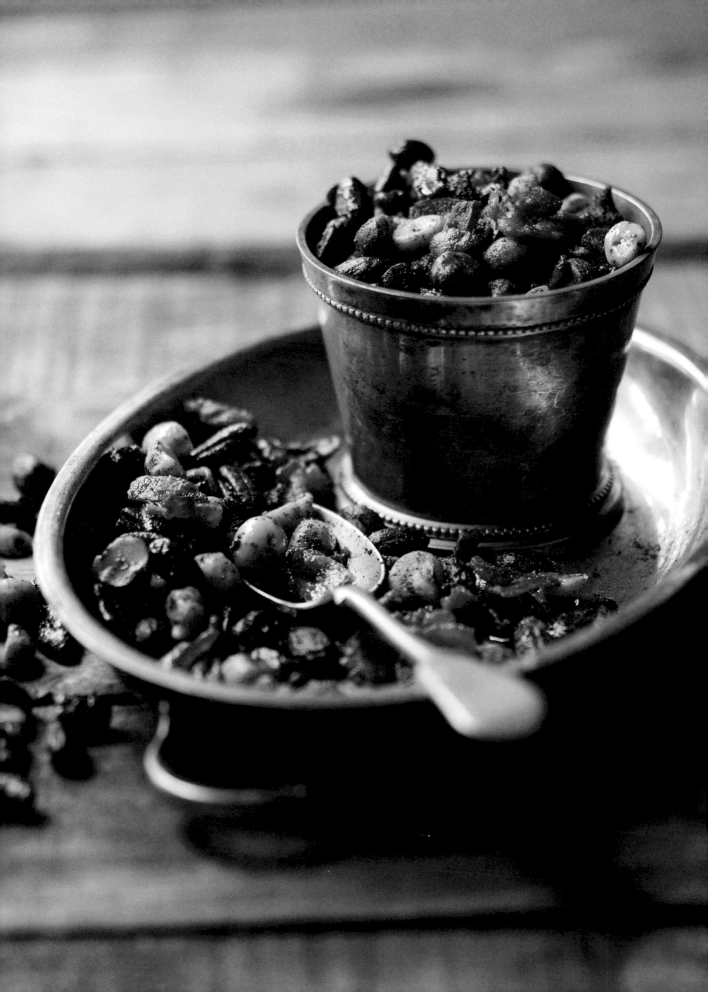

ROASTED COURGETTE HUMMUS

MAKES 500 G

Although chickpeas aren't true carbs, they are quite high in starch which puts them close to the Red List. We've put this one in the 'basics' section because we've found that a dip of some sort is always needed for a quick bite. This is the Greenest dip you're going to get, and it is probably the tastiest too.

500 g courgettes, cut into chunks

Oil or butter for roasting

½ tsp salt, depending on taste

Juice of about 1 large lemon

¼ cup tahini

1 garlic clove, whole

4 tbsp olive oil

Pepper for coating

½ tbsp ground cumin

★ Preheat the oven to 180°C (Gas 4).

★ Toss the courgettes in a light coating of oil or butter, salt and pepper and roast in the oven until golden brown and soft (about 30 to 40 minutes).

★ Place the roasted courgettes in a food processor along with the remaining ingredients and purée until smooth.

★ Leave to infuse for an hour and serve with anything you like.

Note: Using this basic hummus recipe, you can actually swap the chickpeas for quite a few other veggies like pumpkin, butternut squash, aubergine or even sun-dried tomatoes and get a similar, if not better, result.

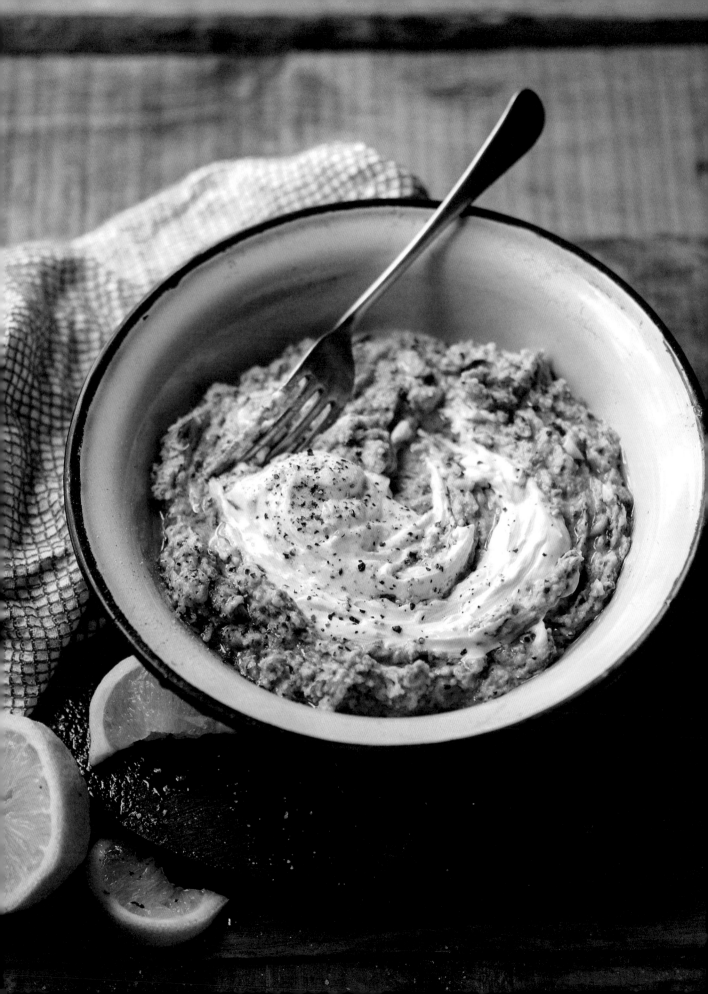

HOT SMOKED FISH PÂTÉ

MAKES 500 G

In South Africa, fish pâté is a staple at any gathering. We use a very bony fish called snoek, which has rich and oily meat and is excellent smoked. Not only is this delicious but it is also a pretty easy way to sneak in some healthy fats and omega 3s during a snack. For this recipe you can use any hot-smoked oily fish as long as it is fresh!

50 g butter

1 large onion, diced

2 garlic cloves, minced

250 g hot-smoked fish (salmon, trout, mackerel, etc.)

100 g cream cheese

100 g crème fraîche

1 handful flat-leaf parsley, roughly chopped

1 tsp paprika

½ tsp cayenne pepper

1 lemon, juiced

★ In a small saucepan, gently cook the onions in the butter until soft and translucent.

★ Add the garlic and cook briefly until fragrant, then remove to cool.

★ In a food processor, blend the fish, cream cheese and crème fraîche until smooth and tip out into a bowl.

★ Add the remaining ingredients and leave to stand for an hour or so to infuse.

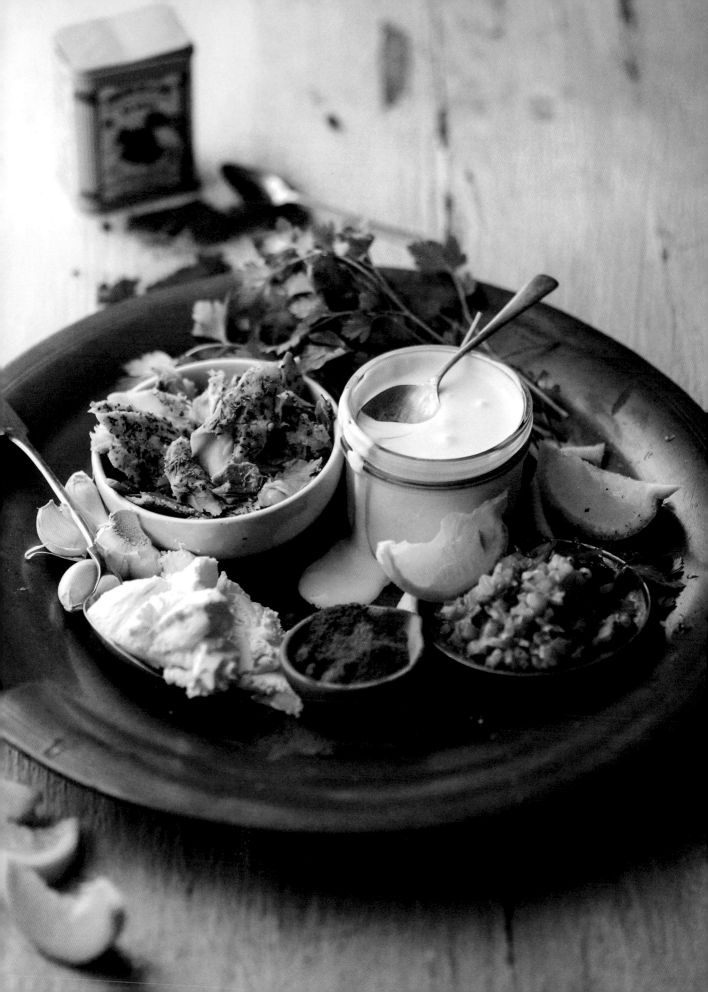

FERMENTED PICKLES

Salted and brined pickles were originally invented to increase the shelf life of food. These days, we just pickle because it tastes good. What we often forget is how good real, homemade natural pickles are for our gut flora. Live bacteria from fermented foods can instantly improve your metabolism and beef up your existing gut flora. Sterilization is often a necessary step in the pickling process, which kills the bacteria. Although this does kill all the good guys, the fermentation process changes the nature of the nutrients into a state that will encourage your probiotic cultures to multiply.

The gherkin is the most popular brined pickle on earth. Before corporates got hold of them and started using vinegar to add fake sourness, all of the acidity came from natural fermentation in a brine solution. Below, we have given you a spice mixture that you can use to pickle just about anything. The brine recipe we've given you uses a 7 per cent salt content. In the colder climates, it is safe to use low-salt brine like a 4 per cent or 5 per cent. Here in Africa, a slightly higher salt content controls the fermentation. It just keeps everything from going a little too wild in the jar. You can use this brine on absolutely any vegetable you would like to pickle.

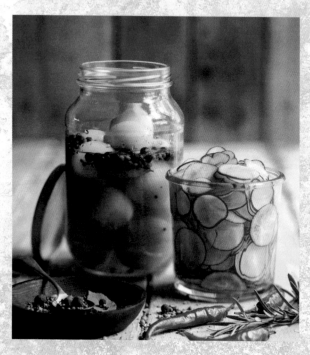

THE BANTING TOOLKIT

FERMENTED PICKLES

1 stick cinnamon, broken up into a few pieces

1 tbsp black peppercorns

1 tbsp yellow mustard seeds

1 tsp fennel seeds

2 tsp whole allspice

2 tsp whole coriander

1 tbsp dill seeds

FOR A BASIC PICKLE

1 l water
Brine

TO PICKLE

1 kg vegetables you wish to pickle – cucumbers, beets, carrots, cauliflower, chillies, garlic

70 g salt (or 7 per cent salt-to-water ratio). Try to use crystal salt; often iodated salt makes the brine go murky.

1 tbsp pickling spice mixture of your choice

1 brined or fresh vine leaf (optional – it will assist in keeping the veggies crunchy)

Brine to cover

TO MAKE FERMENTED PICKLES

★ Combine all of the ingredients and store in a jar.

Note: In all honesty, you could literally use just a teaspoon of mustard seeds. The spice combinations are up to you entirely.

TO PICKLE

★ Clean the vegetables in fresh water and set aside to dry.

★ In a small saucepan, bring the water, salt and spices to the boil. Leave them to cool.

★ Pack the vegetables as tightly as possible into sterilized jars and cover with brine, making sure there is a piece of vine leaf in each jar (again, only optional).

★ Leave them at room temperature for three or four days. Bubbles will begin forming. This is normal; just skim them off and top with more water or brine if you need to.

★ You may need to weigh the veg down with another jar in the beginning to keep them submerged, but once fermentation gets deep into the flesh, they will start sinking.

★ After three weeks, your pickles should be completely finished.

★ You can keep them in the fridge from this point with the lids on. From now on, they will stay edible while they slowly continue fermenting. Store in the fridge an consume within three months

Note: To keep the pickled veg fresher for longer, you can drain them and transfer them to new sterilized jars. Bring the same pickling brine to the boil and pour it back over them in the jars and close.

When they are finished, the veggies should be opaque, crunchy and tart. Slimy, mushy veggies are the result of botched fermentation and are spoilt. Sadly you'll have to throw them away.

The vine leaves are an insurance policy. They help keep the pickles fresh and crunchy. The fermenting brine is hugely nutritious and is said to be an epic hangover cure. Some dried or fresh chilli in the pickling mix would also add a nice kick.

BREAKFAST

Breakfast is where Banting starts on a daily basis. If you can nail a solid fatty breakfast, you have basically won the battle for the day before you leave the house. A good, fatty breakfast will keep you satiated until the mid to late afternoon (provided you don't sneak in that slice of white toast) leaving you with nothing but a light dinner to get through before declaring victory over your carb cravings.

When you're tired and want to do the bare minimum to feed yourself in the morning, it is very hard to muster up the energy to cook something, especially every day. What you will find, though, is that if you do breakfast properly and get the right amount of fat, your energy levels will be a lot more consistent. This is incredibly different from the peaks and troughs you experience after a cereal kick-start. The good news is that after a few weeks of no carbs, you'll find it much easier to get out of bed, light the stove and push on through. Adding to that, if you start your day with a good Green-Listed breakfast, you will stay motivated to stick to Banting for the rest of the day.

Smoked mackerel with avocado and lemon

Kale with chorizo and eggs

Eggs 'baconnaise'

Benchmark omelette

Bacon, asparagus and soft-boiled eggs

Black mushrooms baked in walnut butter
with clotted cream

Bacon-fat cherry tomatoes with bocconcini

'Blitz Ritz' or ripe avocado, cream cheese
and anchovies

Coconut hotcakes and strawberry compôte

Greek yoghurt, almond and strawberry smoothie

Avocado and raspberry shake

Coconut and macadamia frappé

Nut granola

SMOKED MACKEREL WITH AVOCADO AND LEMON

SERVES 2

This is more of a shopping list than a recipe. If you have the ingredients, there's nothing to it.

4 fillets peppered
smoked mackerel

1 ripe avocado

1 lemon

Black pepper

Maldon sea salt

Extra virgin olive oil

★ Just break the mackerel up on a plate. Slice the avocado and scatter it over the mackerel.

★ Squeeze the lemon over it and sprinkle on a good crack of black pepper, a pinch of Maldon salt and a decent splash of oil.

★ If you want to beef it up a little, add a boiled egg or some spring onions or even some rocket.

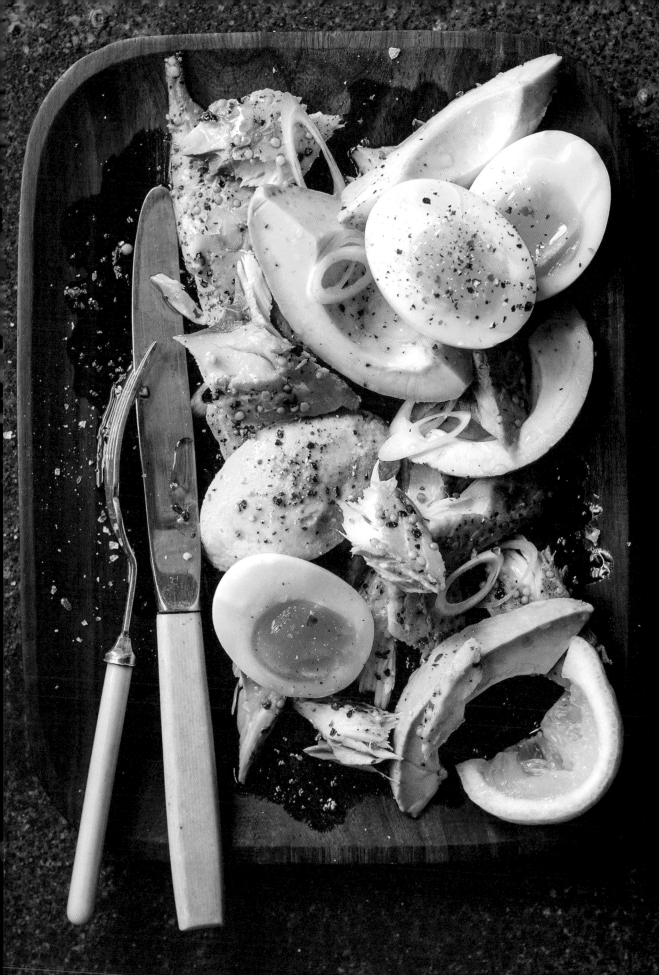

KALE WITH CHORIZO AND EGGS

SERVES 2

Kale has somehow been forgotten about over the last 20 years. It has such a lot to offer nutritionally and is about half the price of spinach, yet hardly anyone knows what to do with it. Because kale is much stronger in flavour than spinach, it needs to be teamed up with big flavour like chorizo or other pungently flavoured ingredients. Having said all of this, you could still easily swap the spinach for kale.

60 g butter

110 g chorizo sausage, thickly sliced

100 g raw kale (or spinach), washed and cut up

¼ cup of water

4 eggs

★ Warm the butter in a heavy-based pan that has a lid. Gently fry the chorizo in the butter until it goes golden brown.

★ Remove the chorizo but keep all the fat and butter in the pan.

★ Crank the heat up to full and fry the kale in the fat until it begins to wilt.

★ Pour the water in and allow it boil ferociously until it is almost fully reduced. If you use a good heavy-based pan and the heat is right this shouldn't take more than a minute.

★ Now shape the kale into four 'nests' in the pan and crack an egg into the middle of each nest. Place the lid on the pan, turn the heat down and cook gently for three minutes.

★ When you remove the lid the eggs should be opaque. Now slide the kale off the pan and garnish with the crispy chorizo.

★ Finally, be sure to pour any excess juices from the pan over each serving.

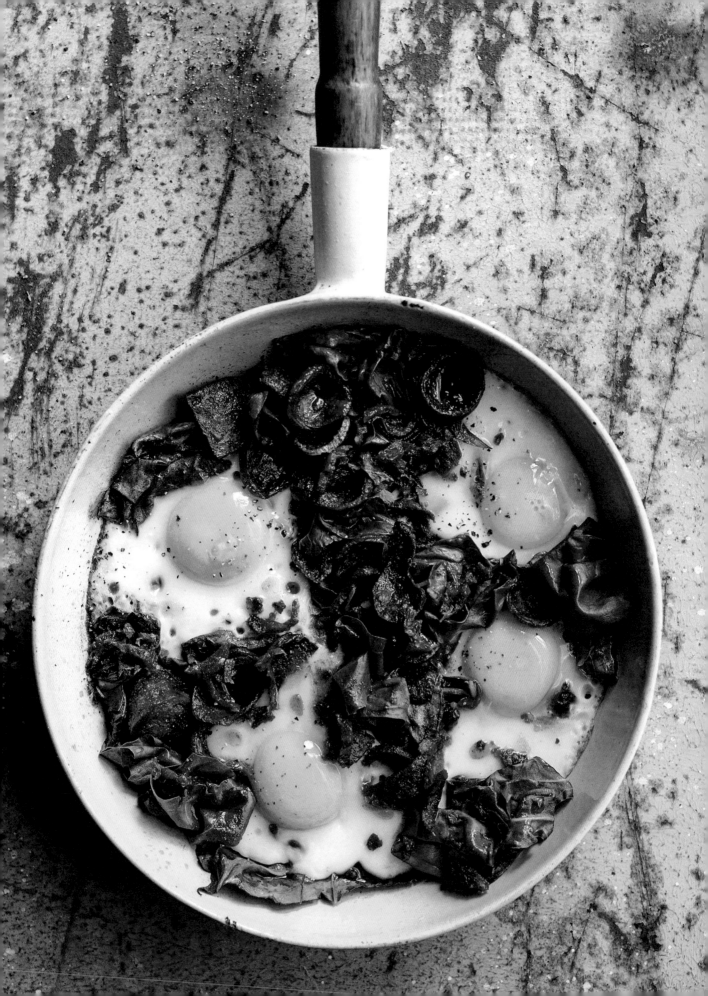

EGGS 'BACONNAISE'

SERVES 2

This is hands-down my favourite breakfast. It's a Banting man's version of Eggs Benedict but in my opinion, it is better. We infuse the bacon into the butter for the hollandaise, giving the hollandaise the most ridiculous smoky bacon flavour – as if hollandaise wasn't already delicious enough. Whoever thought of using bacon fat to make mayonnaise should be knighted. I almost want to repent for all the bacon fat I drained onto paper towels in my previous life. What a terrible waste! This is the perfect breakfast for a special occasion or perhaps a good 'healing' meal on a 'morning after a night before'. I say this because it takes slightly longer than a quick flash in the pan and the methods are slightly more complex. You will need time!

FOR THE ROSTIS

2 small aubergines, grated

1 tbsp table salt

1 egg white

1 tsp psyllium husks

100 g melted butter

FOR THE BACONNAISE

300 g butter

250 g streaky bacon

4 eggs

1 tbsp Dijon mustard

Juice of 1 lemon

Salt and pepper

FOR POACHING

Some vinegar

4 eggs

★ First, make the rostis. Mix the grated aubergine with the table salt and leave it in a sieve for about 30 minutes to drain.

★ Then, using your hands, wring out the aubergine (squeeze quite hard) until it is as dry as possible.

★ Now, mix in the egg white and psyllium and leave for about ten minutes.

★ Then shape the aubergine into large, rosti-shaped cakes.

★ In a heavy-based frying pan, fry the aubergine cakes on a low heat with 100 g of melted butter for about 30 minutes, turning them very carefully every five minutes.

★ Next, make the baconnaise. Place a small saucepan of water on the stove and bring it to the boil.

★ In a large frying pan, fry the bacon on a gentle heat (be careful not to burn the fat or the butter) in 300 g of butter.

★ Once the rashers are crispy, remove from the pan but be sure to leave as much fat as possible back in the pan.

★ Now, separate four eggs, place the yolks, mustard and lemon juice in a heat-proof bowl and place the bowl on top of the saucepan of boiling water (leave it on the heat so it continues to boil).

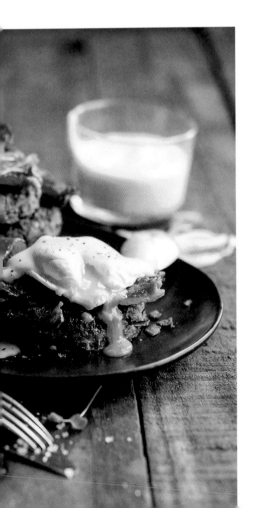

★ Whisk the mixture in the bowl until it becomes light and fluffy.

★ While continuing to whisk, slowly pour in the melted bacon fat and butter mixture. Be careful not to pour it in too fast as it may split.

★ Once you have poured in all of your fat and it has emulsified, your baconnaise is ready. Simply season with salt and pepper and set it aside.

★ Now that the Baconnaise has been set aside, you may use the water in the double boiler to poach the eggs.

★ Season the water with a good splash of vinegar and reduce the heat to a gentle simmer.

★ To poach the eggs, break each one into a small bowl. Now, using a small ladle, swirl the water to create a medium-strength circular current. Then drop the base of the bowl into the centre of the swirl and tip out the egg.

★ Do this one by one with each egg to avoid them cooking into one giant poached egg. Allow them to cook for about three or four minutes (or until soft) then scoop them out using a slotted spoon and drop them onto a paper towel to dab off excess moisture.

★ To serve, place two rostis on each plate and top each rosti with bacon, then a poached egg and finally a massive dollop of baconnaise. Give it a crack of black pepper and dig in.

Note: A tip for the best poached eggs – use the freshest you can find, they hold their shape the best. A tip for making baconnaise or hollandaise – if the mixture gets too thick, add a few drops of hot water. If it starts splitting, do the same and keep whisking. If it splits completely, start again with the lemon, egg yolk and mustard and slowly pour in the split mixture while whisking continuously (as if the split mixture is the butter in the original recipe).

BENCHMARK OMELETTE

MAKES 1

As we mentioned before, a good fatty breakfast will put you on the path to success for a solid day of Banting. The quickest and easiest way to get into the fat first thing in the morning is through a cheesy omelette. If you do this right, you'll be good until dinner time.

2 eggs

80 g any cheese, grated (mature Cheddar is my favourite)

Salt and pepper

A knob of butter

★ Get out of bed and run to the stove.

★ Turn the grill on your oven onto high (so it has time to warm up while you get your other bits together) and place one rack as close to the heating element as possible.

★ Once you've made your coffee, get your eggs together and grate your cheese.

★ Put a small omelette-sized pan onto a fairly high heat.

★ In a small bowl, mix the eggs, salt and pepper with a fork.

★ Add the knob of butter to the pan and the moment it is melted, add in the eggs.

★ Using a wooden spoon or spatula, move the mixture around, exposing as much of the mix as possible to the base of the pan but without leaving any holes.

★ Once the egg has formed a reasonably solid base, but is still very runny on top, cover it with cheese and place the whole pan under the grill.

★ Watch and wait as the eggs puff up and the cheese starts to bubble and melt. The moment your cheese starts going brown and bubbly, remove it from the oven and serve.

Note: The omelette can be filled with absolutely anything. Cheese just happens to be the most cost-effective and easiest to come by. In the South African version of this book we used smoked trout and cream cheese because it sounds fancy, but to be honest not many people rock out the trout at breakfast time. You could use Brie, tomatoes, ham, bacon ... the list goes on. If you find you can't get through a whole omelette, try doing it with only one egg.

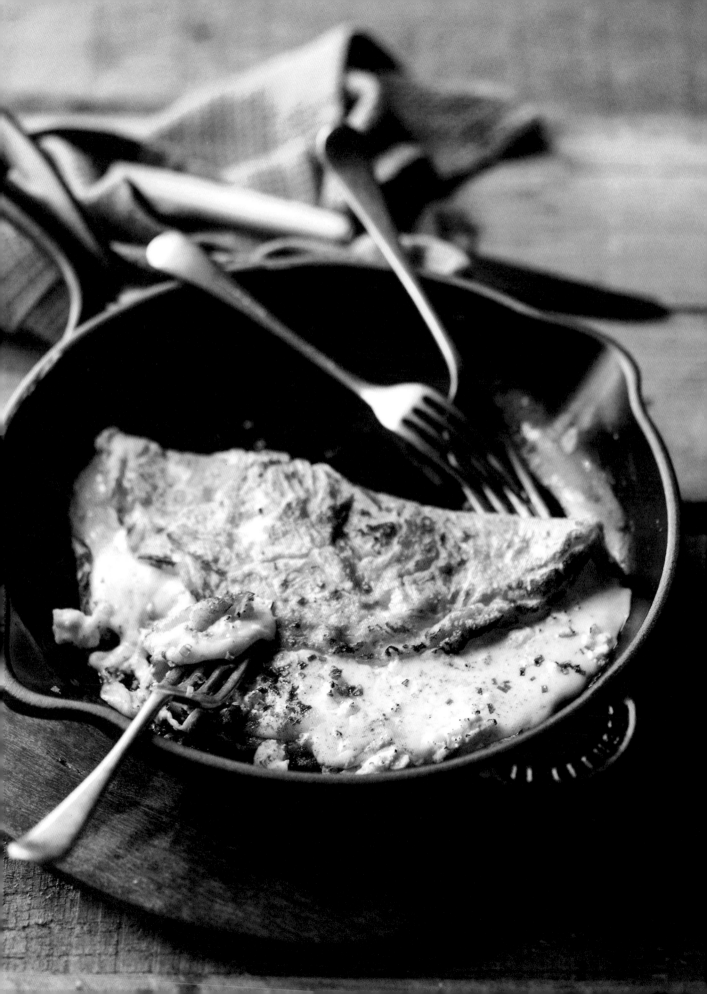

BACON, ASPARAGUS AND SOFT-BOILED EGGS

SERVES 2

250 g streaky bacon

40 g butter

4 eggs

200 g asparagus spears

Salt and black pepper

★ Get a small pot of water on to boil.

★ Fry the bacon in the butter in a heavy-based frying pan until crispy, then remove it from the heat.

★ Drop the eggs into the water (boil for 3.5 minutes for perfect soft-boiled eggs).

★ Blanch the asparagus spears in the egg water for about two minutes. The moment they turn bright green, remove them with tongs and drop them straight into the bacon pan, with the fat and butter and all that other goodness. If the bacon is off the heat already, that's cool.

★ As the eggs come out of the water, turn the bacon and asparagus pan back on and let the asparagus colour a little in the fat.

★ Peel the eggs underwater (it is 1,000 times easier this way).

★ Serve the bacon and asparagus topped with all the pan juices, with the boiled eggs broken over the top and a sprinkle of salt and pepper.

Note: This is a basic warm salad recipe. You can add or take anything away from this. Try swapping the asparagus for mushrooms.

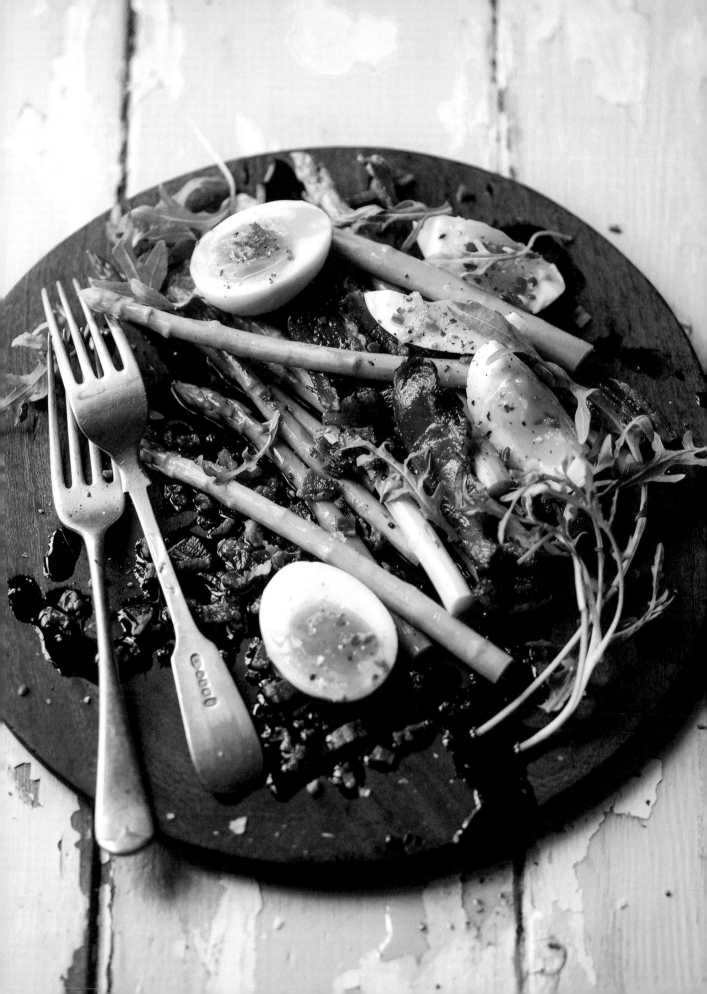

BLACK MUSHROOMS BAKED IN WALNUT BUTTER WITH CLOTTED CREAM

SERVES 2

Another great vegetarian option! You could also use this as a side dish but, for me, the meatiness of those big flat mushrooms is perfect for breakfast. Also, when you're adding that glorious clotted cream at the end, you'll agree that this dish needs nothing else.

4 large flat mushrooms

4 garlic cloves, left whole

1 cup walnuts, gently crushed

120 g butter or lard

120 g clotted cream

Salt and pepper

★ Preheat the oven to 200°C (Gas 6).

★ Lay the mushrooms out on a baking tray and place one clove of garlic in the centre of each one.

★ Mix the walnuts and the butter or lard together and divide the mixture evenly between each mushroom, placing it on top of the garlic.

★ Place the mushrooms in the oven and roast them for about 15 minutes (or until cooked).

★ Serve immediately with a big dollop of the thickest, creamiest clotted cream you can find on each mushroom. Season with salt and pepper.

Note: If you're not a fan of whole cloves of garlic, simply remove them before serving. The flavour will have penetrated right through the mushrooms anyway.

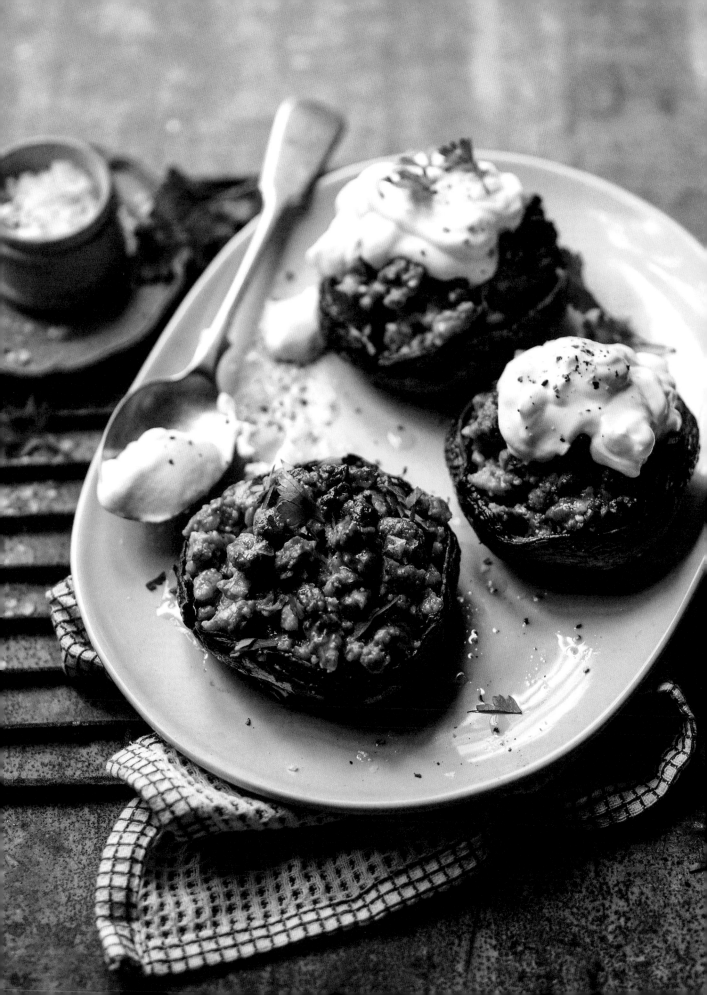

BACON-FAT CHERRY TOMATOES WITH BOCCONCINI

SERVES 4

This is one of those things that you could throw together when you've got leftover cheese from a little salad the night before. Bocconcini are little balls of mozzarella cheese, and they can be found in most supermarkets. Funnily enough, while it's great for breakfast, this dish would also go down a treat at a pizza party where there aren't any carb-free bases.

250 g streaky bacon, cut into 4 cm strips

20 g bacon fat or butter

1 cup large cherry tomatoes

250 g fresh bocconcini (or you can break up a piece of buffalo mozzarella into chunks)

1 handful fresh basil leaves

★ Add the bacon, fat or butter and tomatoes to a cold pan, then place it on the heat.

★ Keep the heat on medium or low for about five minutes to let the fat and juice come out of the bacon. If you want to get a bit more juice out of the tomatoes, you can press down on them gently.

★ Once there are some juices in the pan, crank the heat up to full and stir continuously. The tomatoes should begin colouring and the bacon will start going crispy.

★ Once the tomatoes and bacon are looking brown on the edges, add the cheese and basil and toss them for about 10 seconds, then serve immediately.

Note: Serve this the moment that the cheese starts to melt. If you leave it for any longer the cheese will melt completely and you won't get that amazing sensation of a ball of cheese actually melting in your mouth. If you're fresh out of bocconcini, any cheese will do. Brie and Camembert are superb with tomatoes and melt brilliantly.

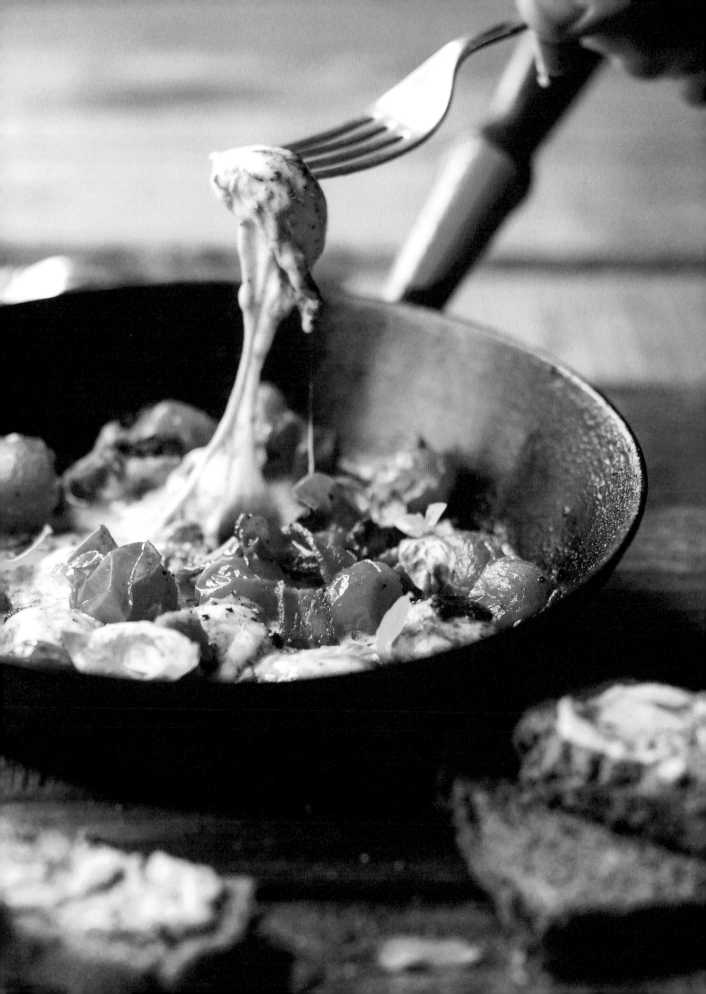

'BLITZ RITZ' OR RIPE AVOCADO, CREAM CHEESE AND ANCHOVIES

SERVES 1

This is a serious on-the-run breakfast. What we love about it is how such a small meal can be packed with so much flavour and fill you up so quickly.

1 large, ripe avocado

2 tbsp heaped, full-fat cream cheese

10 small, top-quality anchovy fillets

½ lemon, juiced

Red or green Tabasco

Cracked black pepper

Extra virgin olive oil (optional)

★ Cut the avocado in half, remove the stone and place the halves on a plate.

★ Top each one with a tablespoon of the cream cheese.

★ Lay the anchovies on top of the cream cheese.

★ Season the whole avocado well with lots of lemon juice, Tabasco sauce, black pepper and even a splash of good peppery extra virgin olive oil if you like.

Note: No need for salt here; the anchovies should be salty enough. The success of this dish depends entirely on the quality of the anchovies. Poor-quality anchovies or pilchards could ruin it, so be discerning and flavour will prevail.

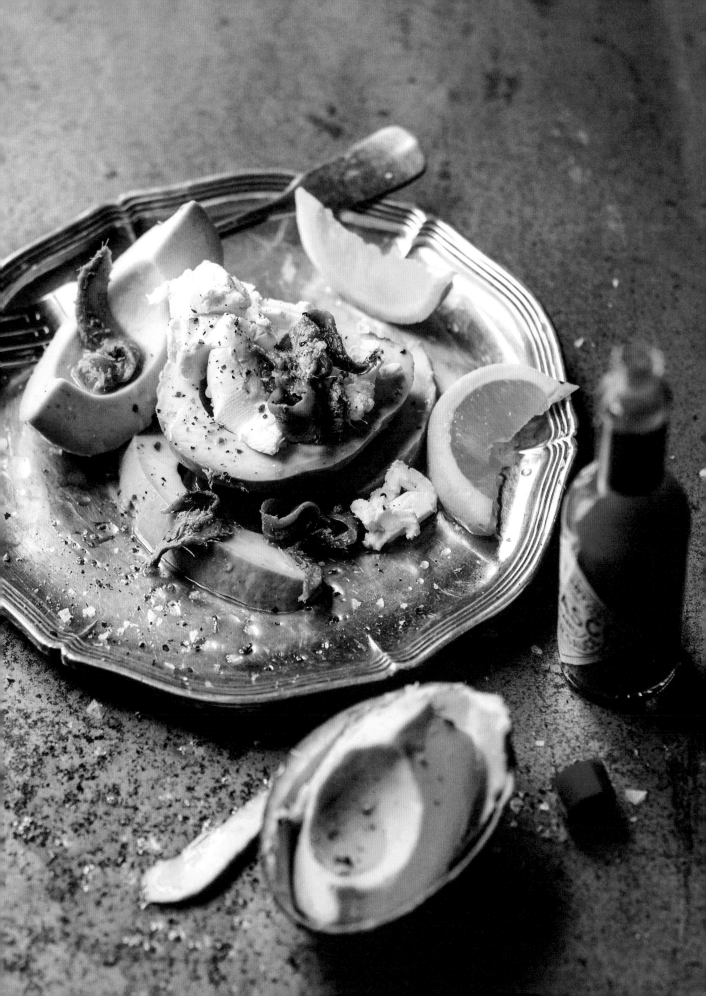

COCONUT HOTCAKES AND STRAWBERRY COMPÔTE

SERVES 4

This particular hotcake, once garnished with the cream cheese, reminds us a lot of our favourite toxic dessert: cheesecake! Fresh berries can be ridiculously expensive, so if you're cooking them, it will make absolutely no difference using frozen ones.

FOR THE HOTCAKES
3 whole eggs, separated

½ cup coconut flour

½ cup almond flour

½ tsp xanthan gum

1 tsp baking powder

2 tsp xylitol

½ tsp vanilla essence

½ cup water

¾ cup coconut milk

3 additional egg whites

Coconut oil for frying

FOR THE COMPÔTE
AND GARNISH
300 g frozen or fresh strawberries, roughly cut

3 tbsp xylitol

200 g full-fat cream cheese

★ Warm the strawberries in a small saucepan on a gentle heat.

★ Once they release their juices add in the xylitol and let them simmer gently for about ten minutes or until slightly softened.

★ Remove from the heat and allow to cool.

★ Whisk all six of the egg whites to the stiff peak stage.

★ Place all of the hotcake ingredients except the egg whites into a bowl and mix them well. Now, gently fold in the egg whites.

★ Get a pan on to a medium heat and add in the coconut oil.

★ Once the oil is warm and melted, drop the hotcake mixture in, one spoonful at a time. Once you see bubbles appearing on the surface, flip them over. Each side should be a light golden brown colour.

★ Top each hotcake with cream cheese and spoon over the strawberry compôte before serving.

Note: If you're not entertaining, don't bother eating them off a plate. We eat these out of the pan. The hotter they are, the softer the cream cheese gets.

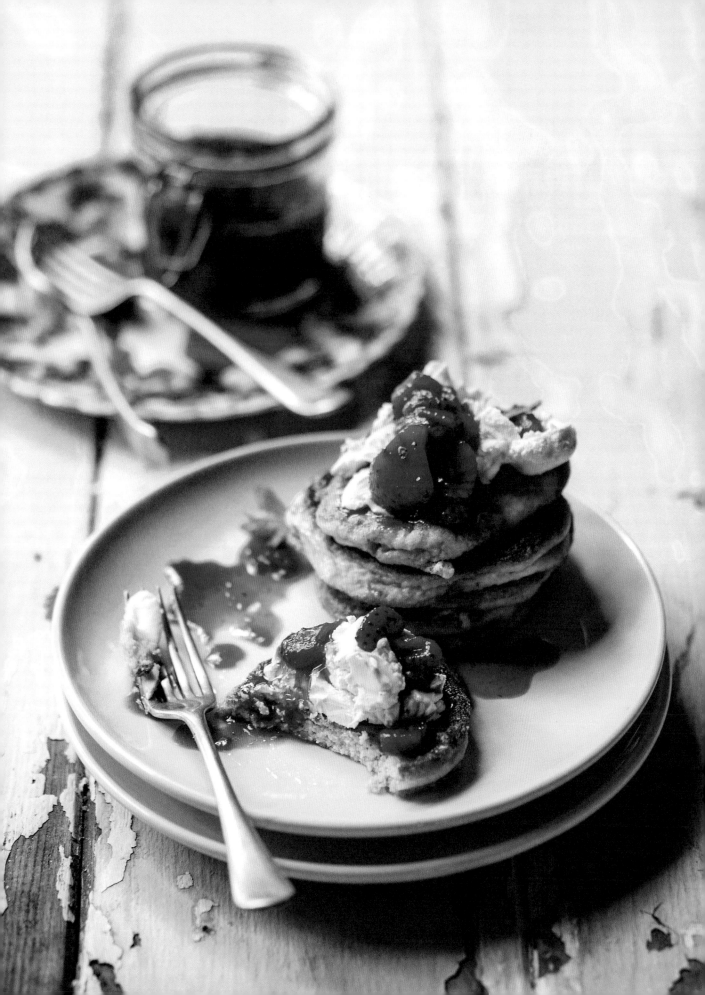

GREEK YOGHURT, ALMOND AND STRAWBERRY SMOOTHIE

MAKES 1

Almonds and strawberries are what we call a 'marriage' of flavours. In this recipe, not only do the flavours complement each other but the texture of the almond butter creates quite a decadent feel. This is by far the quickest breakfast recipe we have, and it's delicious!

3 tbsp almond butter

150 ml extra-thick Greek yoghurt

100 g frozen strawberries

10 ice cubes

1 tsp xylitol (optional)

★ Place all of the ingredients in a food processor or a smoothie machine and blitz. You could also use a stick blender for this too if you prefer.

Note: You should be able to get almond butter in most supermarkets. Alternatively try a health food shop. You could also swap the almond butter for macadamia nut butter if almonds aren't your thing.

AVOCADO AND RASPBERRY SHAKE

MAKES 1

I know, avocado in a shake. Seriously? But the fresh acidity of the raspberries in this shake almost completely masks the avocado flavour, leaving behind only the creamy texture.

½ ripe avocado, peeled and with the stone removed

100 g frozen raspberries

50 g extra-thick Greek yoghurt

50 ml water

A squeeze of lemon juice

½ cup ice cubes

1 tsp xylitol (optional)

★ Combine all the ingredients in a food processor or smoothie machine and blitz.

Note: In all shakes and smoothies where one would usually use banana, we recommend adding avocado instead. Bananas pale in comparison to avocados on the nutritional scale, and to us the texture of avocado is actually smoother.

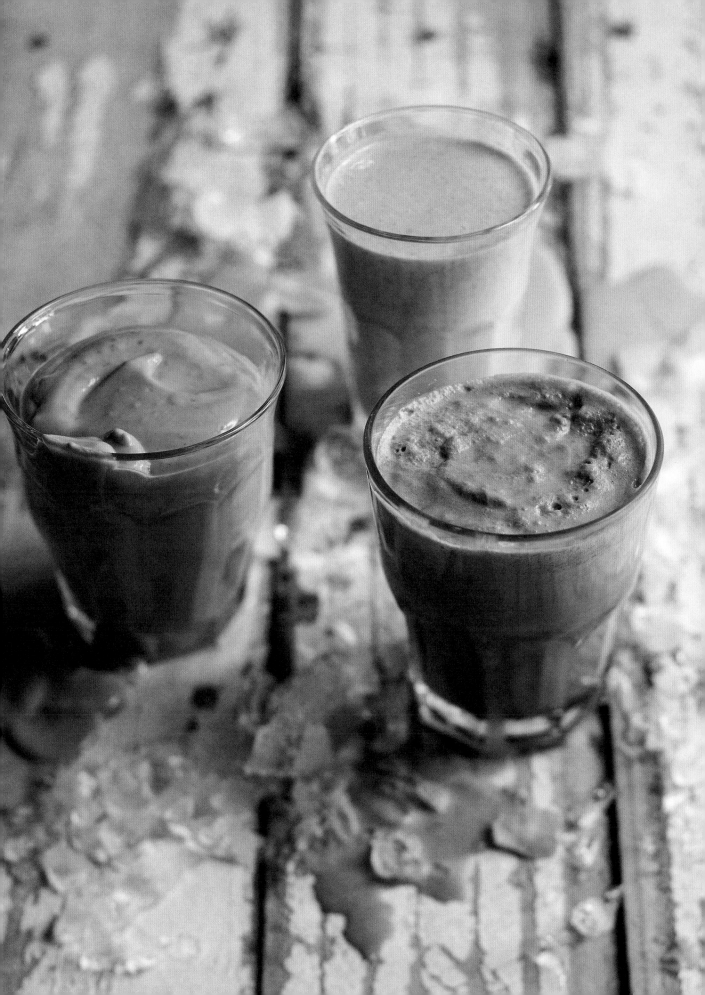

COCONUT AND MACADAMIA FRAPPÉ

MAKES 1

For those who aren't too keen on rich breakfast shakes and fry-ups, this recipe is more like an enriched coffee on the run. It's about as light as a high-fat meal can get but it's better than nothing and it should help crush your hunger, at least until lunch.

1 shot espresso (an extra shot will do no harm if you need a little extra oomph)

½ cup coconut cream

½ cup full cream milk

3 tbsp macadamia nut butter

½ cup ice blocks

1 tsp xylitol (optional)

★ Pour all of the ingredients into a smoothie machine or food processor and blitz until smooth.

Note: You could easily swap the espresso for a teaspoon or two of instant coffee.

NUT GRANOLA

MAKES 12–15 SERVINGS

This 'granola' takes the place of any muesli one might want to have with yoghurt.

100 g walnuts

100 g sunflower seeds

100 g chopped hazelnuts

100 g almond flakes

3 tbsp coconut oil

2 tsp ground cinnamon

2 tsp dried ginger

½ tsp nutmeg

★ Preheat the oven to 160°C (Gas 3).

★ Roughly chop the walnuts and mix together with the sunflower seeds, hazelnuts and almond flakes.

★ Fry the spices in the coconut oil in a large pan, then add the nuts and toast them briefly.

★ Tip the nuts onto an oven tray and bake them for 10 minutes.

★ Cool them on paper towels and store in an airtight container at room temperature for up to 3 weeks.

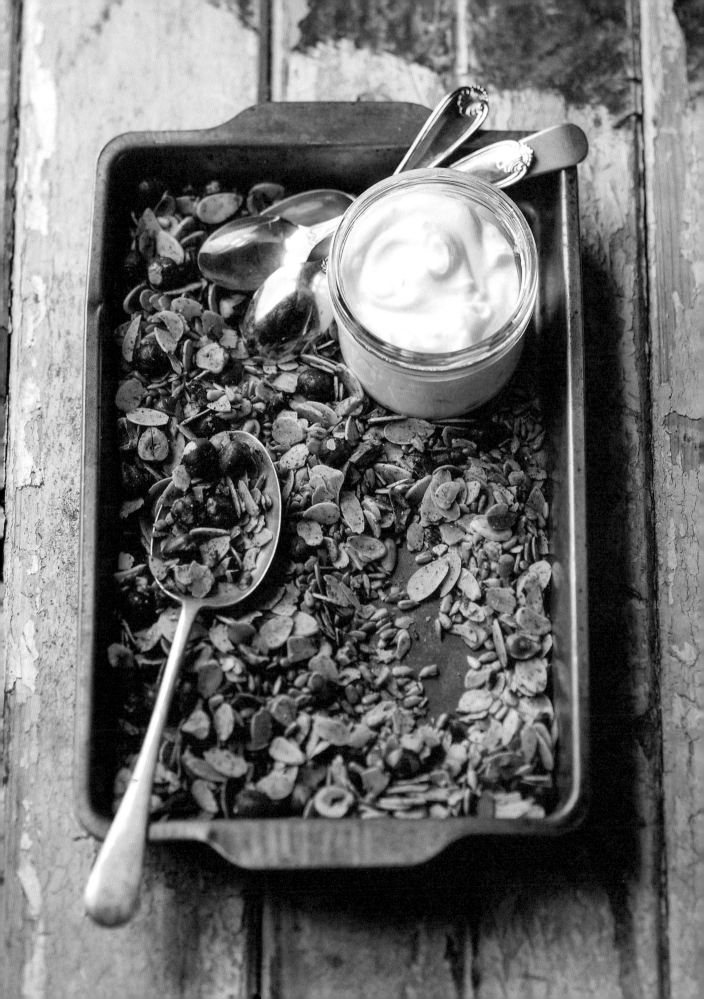

PORK, LAMB AND BEEF

This chapter is, I suppose, what everyone thinks Banting is all about. Lots and lots of meat! I know we've mentioned this in previous chapters, but protein is only a small part of the whole programme. You need the nutrients you can get from meat but please, don't use this chapter as your only lunch and dinner guide as doing so may have an adverse effect on your health.

We have separated sides and meat, poultry and fish dishes to make it easier for people to chop and change side dishes with various proteins. We want you to spend time pairing these recipes with your favourite side dishes. You must eat your veggies!

Lime and sumac rump skewers

Grilled harissa lamb chops with tomato and cucumber salsa

Beef and lime broth

Smoky belly ribs with red slaw

Rosemary salted sirloin with lemon and avocado butter

Quick 'trinchado' on sautéed veg

Fiery beef salad

Beef and cauli-mash cottage pie

Pork larb salad and nouc dressing

Braised short rib

Pork belly, crackling, onions and sage

Rubbed leg of lamb with chimichurri

Lamb blanquette

Green curry pork stir-fry

Lasagne

Smoky pork broth

Carpaccio with Parmesan and capers

Lamb kofta with tzatziki

Bangers and mash

Gammon and mustard cabbage rolls

LIME AND SUMAC RUMP SKEWERS

SERVES 4

This is a great dish for the BBQ. Rump doesn't dry out on the fire as fast as other cuts such as sirloin. It is also much higher in fat, which is what makes it so juicy.

You might not have come across sumac before, but it is available in larger super-markets or from Middle Eastern stores. It has a lemony flavour that is perfect with the lime in this recipe.

480 g beef rump, cut into 20 g cubes

8 skewers (if using bamboo skewers, be sure to soak them in water)

6 garlic cloves, crushed

1 tbsp sumac

3 tbsp extra virgin olive oil

1 tsp salt

1 tsp sesame seeds

1 tsp ground cinnamon

1 tsp ground coriander

1 tsp ground cardamom

1 red onion, cut into big chunks for the kebabs

Large mint leaves

2 limes

★ If using bamboo skewers, soak them in water for at least fifteen minutes.

★ Place all of the ingredients apart from the onion, the mint and limes in a bowl and mix well. If you have time, leave to sit for an hour.

★ Skewer the kebabs with three pieces of meat per skewer, with a sprig of mint and a slice of red onion between each piece of meat.

★ Grill the skewers on the highest heat possible – either on the BBQ or on a griddle pan – until medium rare, then give each one a squeeze of lime and serve immediately.

Note: This is best served with some really thick yoghurt seasoned with lime juice, fresh coriander and chilli.

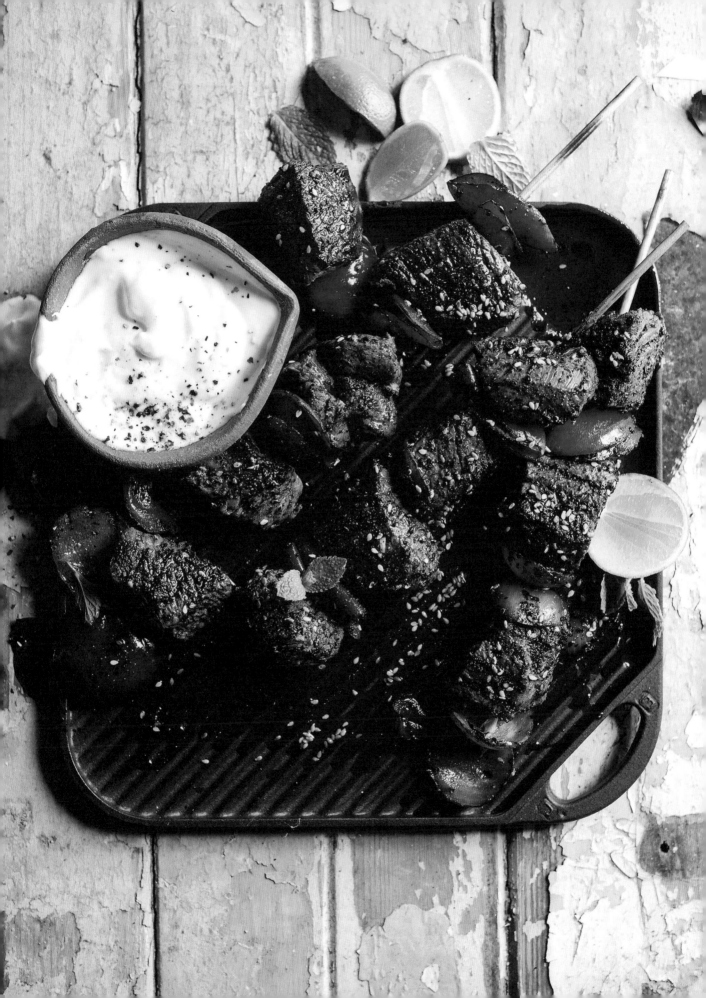

GRILLED HARISSA LAMB CHOPS WITH TOMATO AND CUCUMBER SALSA

SERVES 2

Harissa is a classic North African paste made from chillies and spices. It is usually served with breads, dukkah and olive oil at the beginning of a meal but we use it as a marinade for pretty much anything. Although it does very well on lamb, we also use it on chicken, beef and even vegetables. Mixed with yoghurt, harissa makes a great dip for crudités too.

FOR THE HARISSA PASTE

4 tbsp coconut oil

1 tbsp chopped garlic

1 tbsp deseeded and chopped red chilli

1 tsp ground caraway seeds

2 tsp ground cumin

1 tsp ground coriander

50 g tomato paste (purée)

A little olive oil for drizzling

1 tbsp sweet paprika

1 handful fresh coriander

1 tsp salt

FOR THE LAMB CHOPS

2 lamb chops, about 3 cm thick

1 batch harissa paste (see above)

★ For the harissa, melt the coconut oil in a small saucepan or frying pan. Once the coconut oil is warm but not too hot, add the garlic, chilli, caraway, cumin, coriander and salt.

★ Gently fry the ingredients in the oil until they become fragrant (probably about three or four minutes).

★ Add in the tomato paste and sauté it gently for a few more minutes.

★ Remove from the heat and scrape the contents of the pan into a narrow container (the jug that comes standard with a stick blender is a great option).

★ Now, add to this mixture the paprika and the fresh coriander and blend with a stick blender.

★ Drizzle a little bit of olive oil on top to keep fresh. It should keep for a month in the fridge.

★ For the lamb chops, rub the harissa paste on both sides of the meat and leave to marinate for at least an hour in the fridge.

★ Remove from the fridge and allow the chops to come to room temperature (about 20 minutes).

★ Heat a griddle pan over high heat until almost smoking, then place the chops on the griddle pan, fat side down (on their backs) to start with in order to crisp up the fat nicely.

FOR THE TOMATO AND CUCUMBER SALSA

2 large, firm tomatoes, finely chopped

½ cucumber, finely diced

½ small red onion, finely chopped

Juice of one lemon or lime

4 tbsp extra virgin olive oil

1 handful mint, roughly chopped

1 garlic clove, minced

Salt and pepper

★ Once the fat is nicely crisped, turn them on to their sides and sear for about 2 minutes.

★ Flip the chops over and cook for another 3 minutes for medium-rare and 3½ minutes for medium. Remove from the heat and let them rest before serving with delicious salsa.

★ To make the tomato and cucumber salsa, combine all the ingredients together and leave to stand for at least 20 minutes to allow the flavours to infuse.

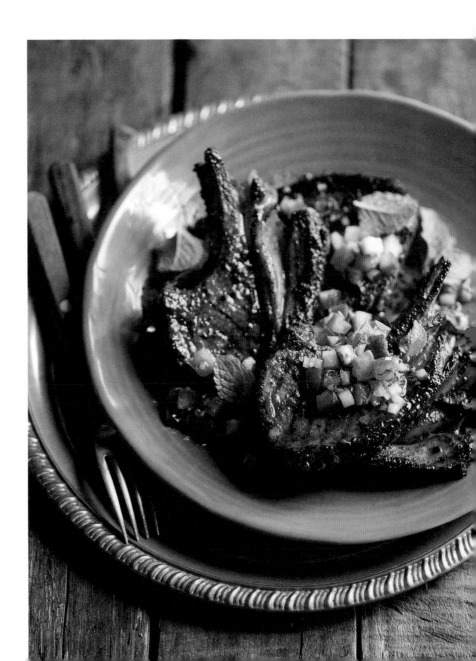

BEEF AND LIME BROTH

SERVES 4

As mentioned earlier, broths are the only way for us to get valuable nutrients and minerals out of the bones of animals. Eating plain old broth is a bit dull so this recipe is just one idea we have that will spice up your basic broth recipe.

Oil or butter for frying

1 large red chilli, deseeded and roughly chopped

2 tbsp sweet paprika

1.2 l rich beef stock

1 large onion, sliced

2 garlic cloves, minced

2 large tomatoes cut into 6 wedges each

160 g green beans, topped, tailed and cut in half

100 g baby spinach

Juice of 2 limes

1 small handful mint

Salt and pepper

★ In a splash of oil or a little butter, sauté the onions until soft. Add the garlic and stir until fragrant.

★ Add the stock and bring to the boil.

★ Now add the tomatoes, chilli and paprika and boil until the flavours have combined nicely. This may take about ten minutes.

★ Add in the green beans and simmer until they turn bright green. Finally, add the spinach, the mint and lime juice.

★ Season to taste with salt and pepper and serve.

Note: Some seared steak pieces would 'beef' this up if you wanted to have it as a main meal.

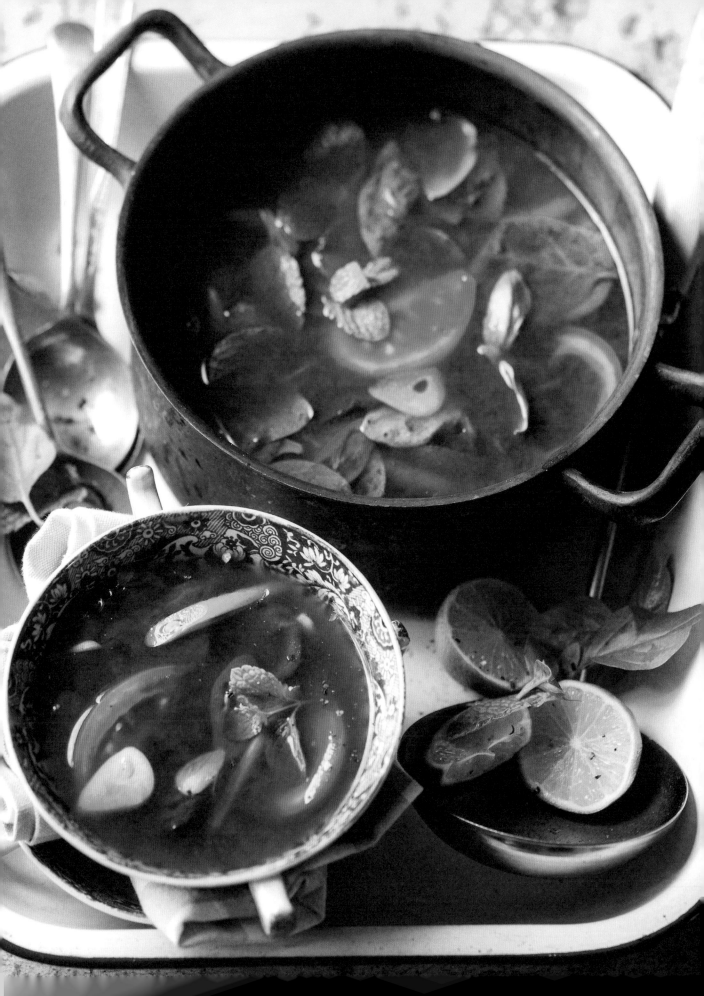

SMOKY BELLY RIBS WITH RED SLAW

SERVES 4

After a lot of research, we found that sugar-free pork rib recipes are almost non-existent. But pork ribs (smoked ribs especially) are one of the most delicious things out there. You need a sugar-free rib if you ever want a BBQ to be the same again, and we've found one! Garnish these with a twist of lime and a sprinkle of cayenne pepper.

FOR THE BELLY RIBS

2.4 kg belly ribs

2 cups saved cooking juices, broth or stock (chicken or pork)

100 g can tomato paste

¼ cup apple cider vinegar

¼ cup Dijon mustard

1 tsp ground cumin

2 tsp sea salt

4 tbsp xylitol

2 tsp smoked paprika

2 tsp dried oregano

Black pepper to taste

FOR THE RED SLAW

½ red cabbage

½ red onion, finely sliced

1 tsp English mustard

1 tbsp apple cider vinegar

1 tbsp creamed horseradish

¼ cup Banting Mayonnaise (see page 66)

2 tbsp crème fraîche

★ Preheat the oven to 180°C (Gas 4).

★ Combine all of the ingredients in a deep tray, being sure to lay the ribs out flat. If they are not fully submerged, top up the tray with some water.

★ Cover the tray with foil and bake for 2 hours.

★ Remove the ribs from the heat and leave them to cool for a while in their juices. Once cool, strain the liquid into a pot and simmer until it has reduced down to a sticky glaze.

★ Grill or BBQ the ribs while basting them constantly with the glaze on both sides.

★ When they start to go black at the edges, remove them from the heat, cut them up and enjoy.

★ To make the slaw, simply mix all of the ingredients well in a large bowl and serve.

Note: This can be done with loin/back ribs too. You could also reduce these ingredients down without the ribs and use the glaze to baste anything on the BBQ.

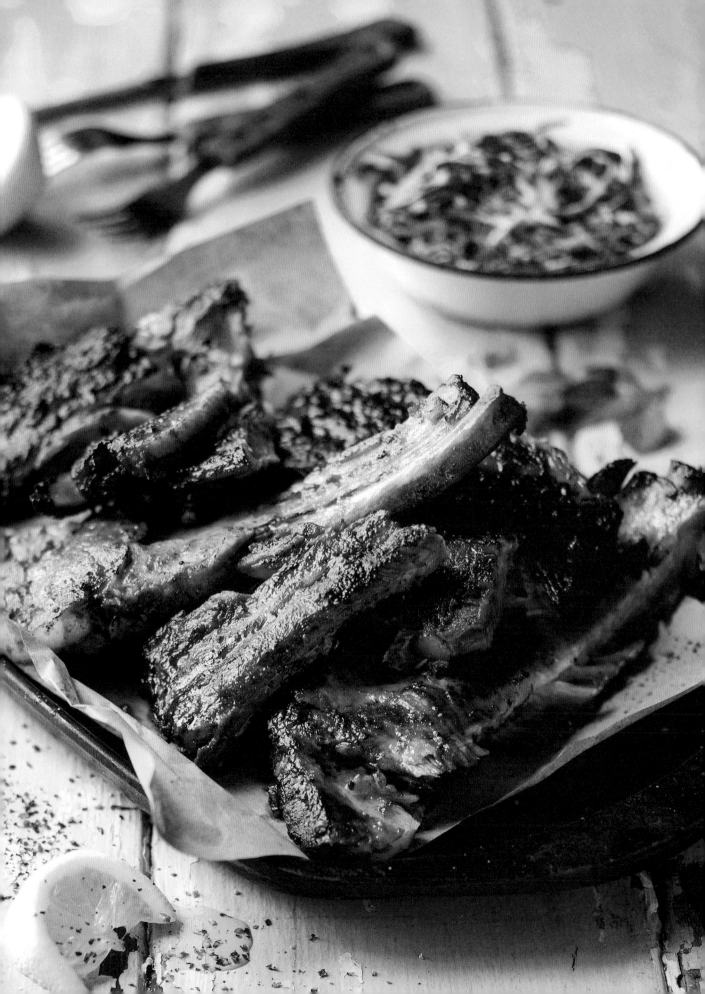

ROSEMARY SALTED SIRLOIN WITH LEMON AND AVOCADO BUTTER

SERVES 2

This is one of the most delicious ways to get extra fats and avocado is probably the most delicious fat you can get. This recipe is inspired by Jonno's first head chef, Mike, who taught him the art of avocado hollandaise – true story.

FOR THE AVOCADO BUTTER

1 large soft ripe avocado

80 g butter at room temperature

2 tbsp cream cheese

1 red chilli, deseeded and finely chopped

1 big handful fresh coriander, roughly chopped

Finely chopped zest and juice of a big, juicy lemon

Black pepper

FOR THE STEAK

2 x 180 g well-aged, fatty and delicious sirloin steaks

1 tsp dried rosemary (or really finely chopped fresh rosemary)

½ tsp roughly ground coriander seeds

½ tsp crystal salt

½ tsp black peppercorns, cracked

¼ tsp chilli flakes

★ First, make the avocado butter. Combine the avocado, butter and cream cheese in a food processor and blend until smooth. Remove the mix from the blender and stir in the remaining ingredients. Store in the fridge in an airtight container.

★ For the steaks, mix all of the rub ingredients together and sprinkle them liberally onto both sides.

★ Get a griddle pan seriously hot – get it smoking.

★ Push the steaks together, side by side, so that they can be stood up on their fat, then grill them fat side down.

★ Once the fat has crisped up and they have rendered a bit of fat into the pan, turn the steaks to grill on their sides.

★ Grill each side for about two or three minutes then rest them away from the heat before serving with the butter.

Note: To go the extra mile, place a fat pat of butter on top of each steak and give it a flash under a grill to soften the butter up.

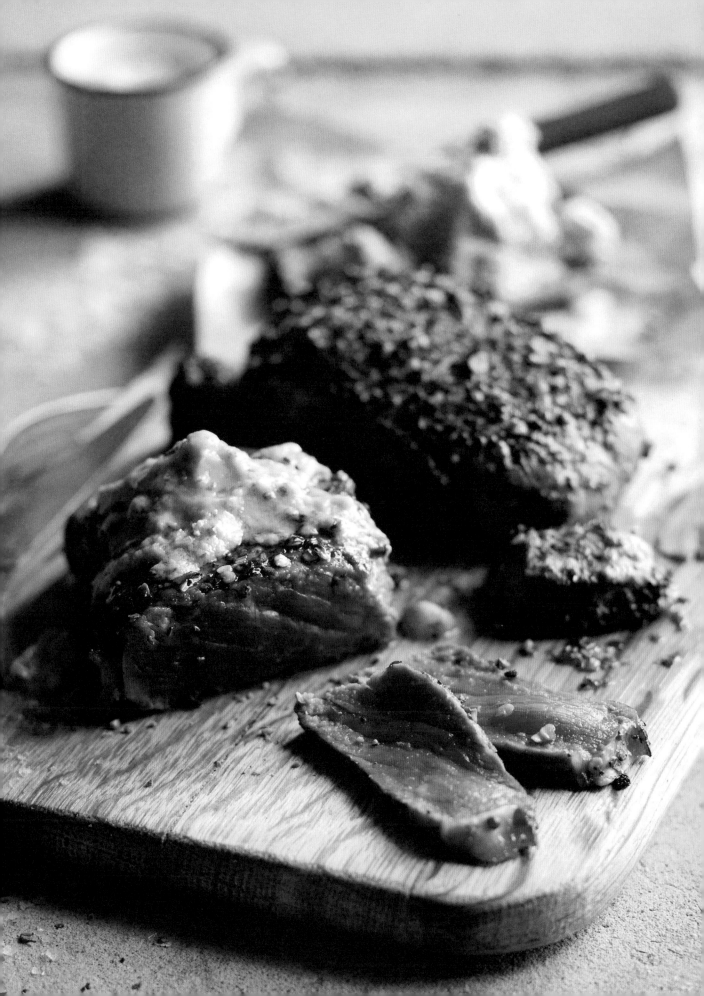

QUICK 'TRINCHADO' ON SAUTÉED VEG

SERVES 4

Trinchado, a rich garlic and chilli-flavoured stew, was one of my favourite snacks in my restaurant days. Unbeknown to the boss, any beef offcuts we couldn't serve would go into the daily trinchado lunch, which became a small competition among the chefs. If only I'd had this recipe back then, I might have won it once or twice.

400 g rump steak, cut into 25 g cubes

A little oil and seasoning

50 g butter

1 large red onion, roughly chopped

1 tbsp garlic and chilli paste (any good quality one)

1 cup green olives, pitted if possible

1 cup beef stock

Juice of one lemon

1 tsp smoked paprika (preferably hot)

1 large handful flat-leaf parsley, roughly chopped

FOR THE SAUTÉED VEG

40 g butter

1 large red onion, sliced

2 red peppers, deseeded and sliced

1 yellow pepper, deseeded and sliced

4 small courgettes cut into quarters, lengthways

3 tbsp capers

★ Get a large heavy-based pan smoking hot.

★ Oil and season the beef cubes well. Tip them into the pan and leave to colour without moving them.

★ Once they have coloured on one side, use tongs to flip them over to colour on another side. If you move them around too much, they will not colour as well and will release too many juices. You may need to do this in two batches to prevent the juices coming out of the meat.

★ Before the meat gets to medium-rare (2 minutes) tip the meat into a tray and cool.

★ Using the same hot pan, without cleaning it, add the butter and the onions and sauté until golden brown.

★ Now add the garlic and chilli paste and sauté until it becomes aromatic.

★ Add the olives, beef stock, lemon juice and smoked paprika and boil until the sauce is reduced by half.

★ Just before serving, add the parsley and tip the meat back in to warm through to medium rare/medium before serving.

★ Serve immediately with the sautéed veg: melt some butter in a medium-sized frying pan, add the onions, peppers and courgettes and sauté them until they soften. Finally, add the capers and mix them through before serving.

Note: For a little extra smokiness we often add some sliced chorizo to the sautéed veg!

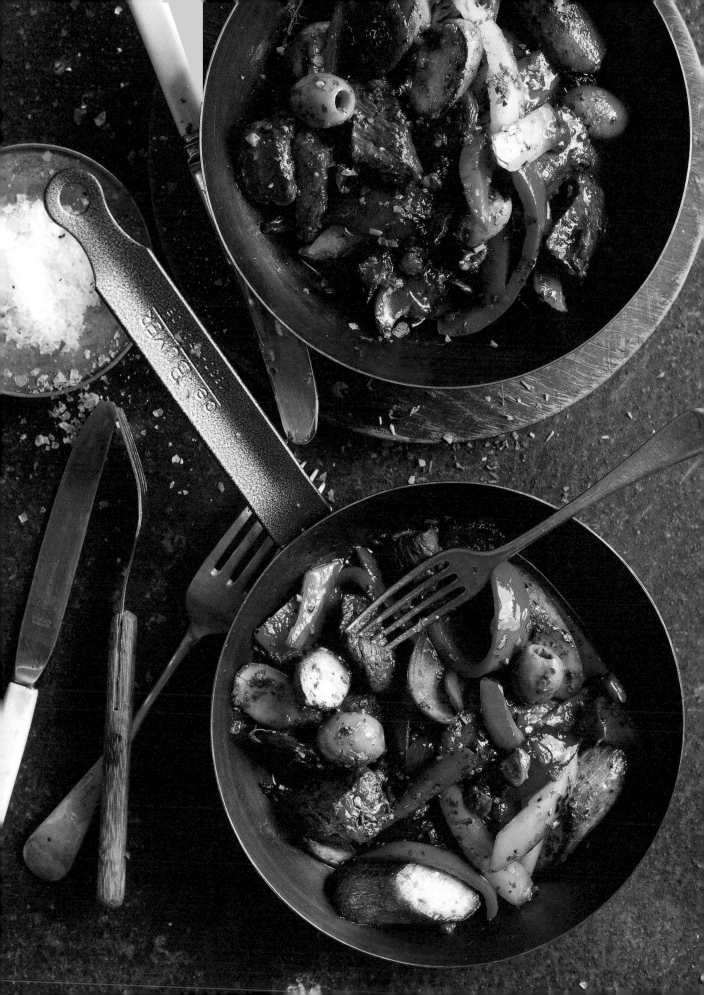

FIERY BEEF SALAD

SERVES 4

Imagine sipping a cocktail with your feet in the sand while you get a really good back massage. This salad will give you a similar feeling of bliss.

FOR THE DRESSING

The juice of two limes

1 handful fresh coriander, roughly chopped

1 tbsp water

1 tbsp Thai fish sauce

1 garlic clove, minced

1 tsp good strong chilli paste

½ stick lemongrass, finely chopped

1 knob (about thumb-sized) ginger, finely grated

FOR THE SALAD

500 g fillet steak

Salt and pepper for seasoning

Splash of oil

4 small heads butterhead lettuce

100 g cherry tomatoes, quartered

100 g beansprouts

½ cucumber, julienned

5 spring onions, julienned

1 big handful mint leaves

1 big handful fresh basil, very roughly chopped

4 tbsp toasted sesame seeds

★ First, make the dressing by simply combining all of the ingredients and leave in the fridge to infuse for up to an hour.

★ Place a griddle pan on the heat and get it smoking hot.

★ Season the steak liberally with salt and pepper and a splash of oil.

★ Drop the steak into the griddle pan and allow a good brown crust to form on the outside. You'll probably need about three or four minutes on each side for this (four sides).

★ Once you have reached that dark colour and the beef is cooked to your liking, remove the steak from the pan and let it rest for about five minutes.

★ Slice the steak as thinly as possible then assemble the salad ingredients.

★ Finally, just before serving, drench the salad in the dressing and tuck in.

Note: This salad would also be great with chicken instead of beef.

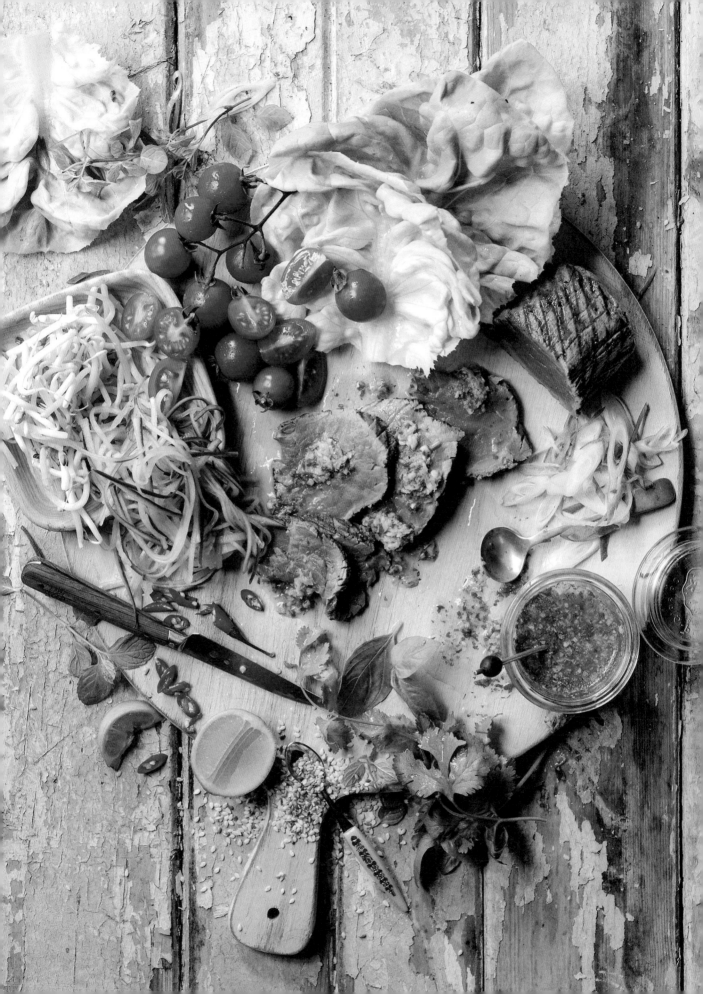

BEEF AND CAULI-MASH COTTAGE PIE

SERVES 6

Like lasagne, cottage pie is a staple on the home-cooked meal roster. With potatoes out of the picture we can make a quick adjustment and use cauliflower to make that delicious crusty topping.

FOR THE MINCE

800 g beef mince

2 tbsp butter

1 large onion, finely chopped

1 stick celery, finely chopped

2 garlic cloves, finely chopped

1 tin (400 g) whole peeled tomatoes, chopped

1 cup beef stock

1 bay leaf

4 tbsp Worcestershire sauce

1 handful fresh basil, roughly chopped

FOR THE CAULI-MASH

1 head cauliflower, broken into florets

2 egg yolks

100 g butter

Salt and pepper

1 pinch ground nutmeg

★ Preheat oven to 190°C (Gas 5).

★ Fry the mince in the butter in a large saucepan until it is golden brown, breaking it up as finely as you can with the wooden spoon.

★ Remove from the pan, add the onions and celery to the same pan and fry them on a medium heat until they go soft. Now add the garlic and sauté until it becomes aromatic.

★ Add the rest of the ingredients, returning the mince to the pan, and mix everything together.

★ Turn the heat down to low and leave it to simmer for half an hour. Stir every now and then to make sure it doesn't stick.

★ While the sauce is cooking, make the cauli-mash. Steam the cauliflower until soft, then drain off any excess moisture.

★ Place the cauliflower in a food processor and purée until smooth.

★ While the blender is running, add in the egg yolks and the butter and continue blending until the butter is melted and well incorporated.

★ Season to taste with salt, pepper and nutmeg.

★ To assemble, fill a lasagne/pie dish with the mince and smooth it out. Top it with the cauli-mash and smooth out again. Place under the grill for 15 minutes until golden brown.

Note: You can add anything exciting to the mince that you think will add to the flavour! If you need a little extra fat, I would recommend giving the crust a generous sprinkling of cheese.

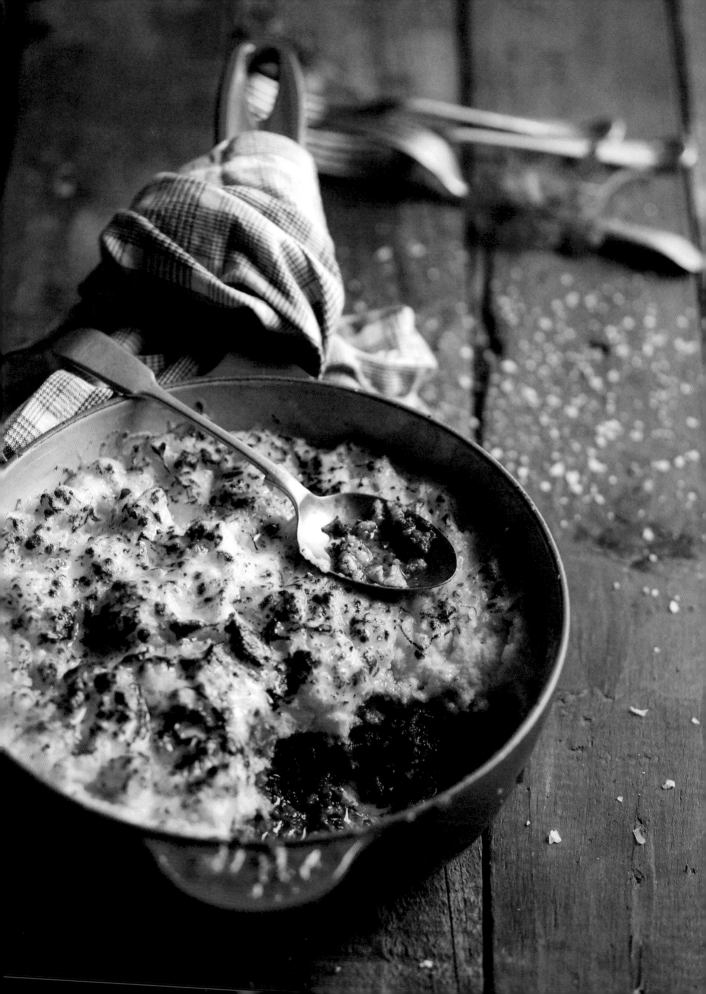

PORK LARB SALAD AND NOUC DRESSING

SERVES 2

This is a traditional dish that I had over in Thailand a few years ago. It's a real winner.

FOR THE PORK

400 g fatty pork mince
(at least 20 per cent fat)

1 tbsp garlic, finely chopped

1 tbsp ginger, finely chopped

1 tbsp chilli paste

½ stick lemongrass, grated
or finely chopped

1 tsp Chinese five spice
powder

¼ tsp ground cardamom

1 small bunch spring onions,
finely sliced

1 tbsp fish sauce

Juice of one lime

½ handful fresh coriander,
roughly chopped

½ handful fresh basil,
roughly chopped

4 large cos or iceberg lettuce
leaves

FOR THE NOUC DRESSING

1 tbsp lemon juice

1 tbsp apple cider vinegar

1 tbsp water

4 tbsp xylitol

4 tbsp fish sauce

1 red chilli, deseeded and sliced

1 garlic clove, chopped

★ In a large, heavy-based pan, fry the mince in its own fat until golden brown.

★ Once the mince is golden brown, add the chilli paste, lemongrass, Chinese five spice and cardamom and fry again until dark brown.

★ Finally, add the spring onions, fish sauce, lime juice, fresh coriander and basil and stir for a minute.

★ Pile the pork mince into the lettuce leaves, using the leaves like taco shells. Combine all the dressing ingredients together, stirring until the xylitol is dissolved, and splash liberally over the pork.

Note: Make sure you get really sweet, fresh, plump, crunchy lettuce for best results.

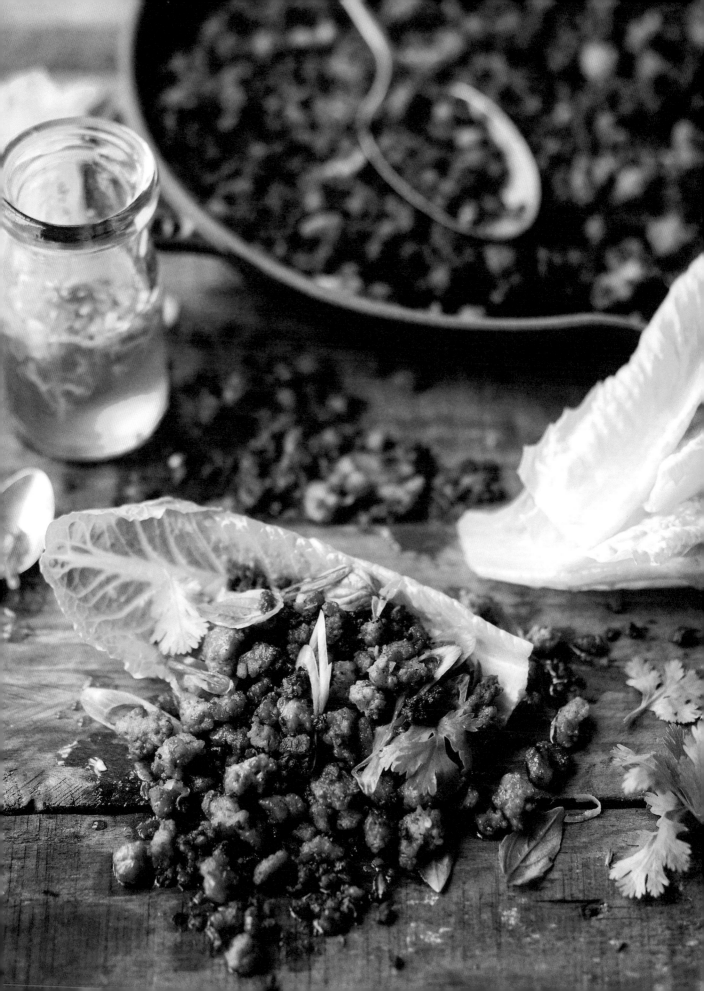

BRAISED SHORT RIB

SERVES 4

To get this recipe right, you will need to visit your butcher. Ask him or her to cut the ribs across the bones into 4 cm-thick sections. Remember that with short ribs, slow and steady wins the race.

½ tbsp coriander seeds

½ tbsp cumin seeds

½ tsp cracked black pepper

1 onion, cut into quarters

1 apple, cut into quarters

2 garlic cloves, cut in half

1 big sprig rosemary

2 tbsp xylitol

½ tbsp fine salt

¼ tsp cayenne pepper

2 racks beef ribs (each cut in half)

Zest of 1 large orange, thickly sliced

2 cups beef broth or stock

½ cup red wine

★ Preheat your oven to 150°C (Gas 2).

★ In a dry frying pan, toast the coriander, cumin and black pepper, then lightly grind them in a pestle and mortar.

★ Spread the onion, apple and garlic onto an oiled baking tray. Pack the four beef rib pieces tightly onto the bed of onion and apple, leaving as little space as possible between them.

★ Now, sprinkle the spices rosemary, xylitol, salt, cayenne pepper and the orange zest over the meat and cover everything in the tray with stock and the wine.

★ The meat should be fully submerged – if not, top it up with a little water.

★ Cover the tray tightly with tin foil and place it in the oven for three and a half hours.

★ After three hours, remove the tray from the oven and leave it to cool, still covered, for 30 minutes.

★ Strain the liquid from the tray into a small saucepan and simmer the juices down to a syrup.

★ Turn the grill on to a high setting, baste the ribs with the syrup and char them under the grill until they get those delicious sticky black bits. Serve with whatever veg you like – we would recommend some Red Slaw (see page 124) or for those who are less 'Green List' perhaps even some sweet potato wedges.

Note: Be careful – these ribs are incredibly delicate once they are cooked.

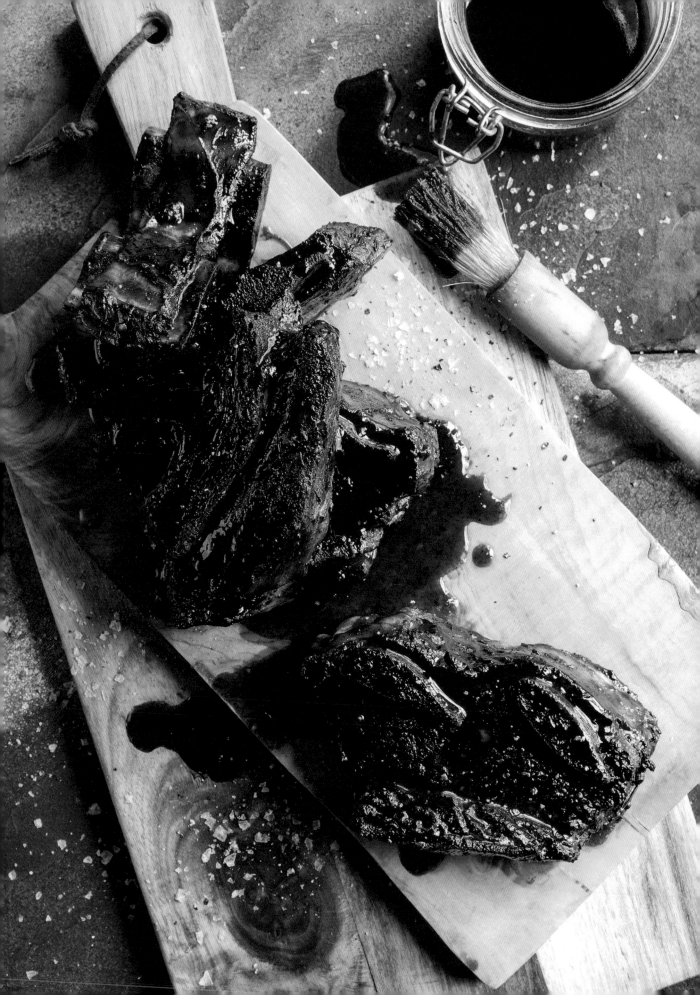

PORK BELLY, CRACKLING, ONIONS AND SAGE

SERVES 4-6

Pork, salt and fennel! Like Snap, Crackle and Pop, they belong together.

FOR THE BELLY

1.2 kg pork belly (bones out, skin on, unrolled)

3 tbsp melted coconut oil

1 tsp fine salt

1 tbsp coarse salt

1 tbsp whole fennel seeds

FOR THE ROASTED ONIONS

40 g butter

4 onions, skin on, cut in half from root to stem

3 fresh bay leaves, torn

Large handful torn sage leaves

★ Preheat the oven to 160°C (Gas 3).

★ Pat the pork belly dry with paper towel then massage the coconut oil and fine salt into the skin, giving it a good coating – with this recipe, we don't score the fat.

★ Now, sprinkle both sides with the coarse salt and fennel seeds, patting them to make sure they stick.

★ Put a roasting rack into a medium-depth oven tray and place the pork on the rack, skin side up. Add three or four cups of water to the tray (making sure   the water doesn't touch the pork) and place the tray on the bottom rack in the oven, leaving it to roast for 1½–2 hours.

★ While the belly is roasting, get a heavy-based, ovenproof frying pan on the heat. Melt the butter and add the onions, skin sides up. Let them simmer in the butter for about ten minutes until they start to go brown and the butter turns nutty. Add the bay and sage to the pan and place in the oven with the pork belly for about an hour.

★ After 1½ hours, check to see if the crackling is very crispy. If not, give it another 30 minutes (you might need to add an extra splash of water).

★ Check again after 30 minutes and if necessary crank the heat up to 200°C (Gas 6) and leave the pork in the oven for another 20 minutes. You will achieve crackling success but you may need to keep an eye on it.

★ Once the belly is done, drain the juices from the tray into a small saucepan and reduce to a rich gravy (depending on the amount of water you put in, you may not need to reduce this). You could add anything from mustard to some fine herbs to give this light gravy a little more depth.

Note: This will also go very nicely with 'cauli-mash' (page 68) and/or braised fennel.

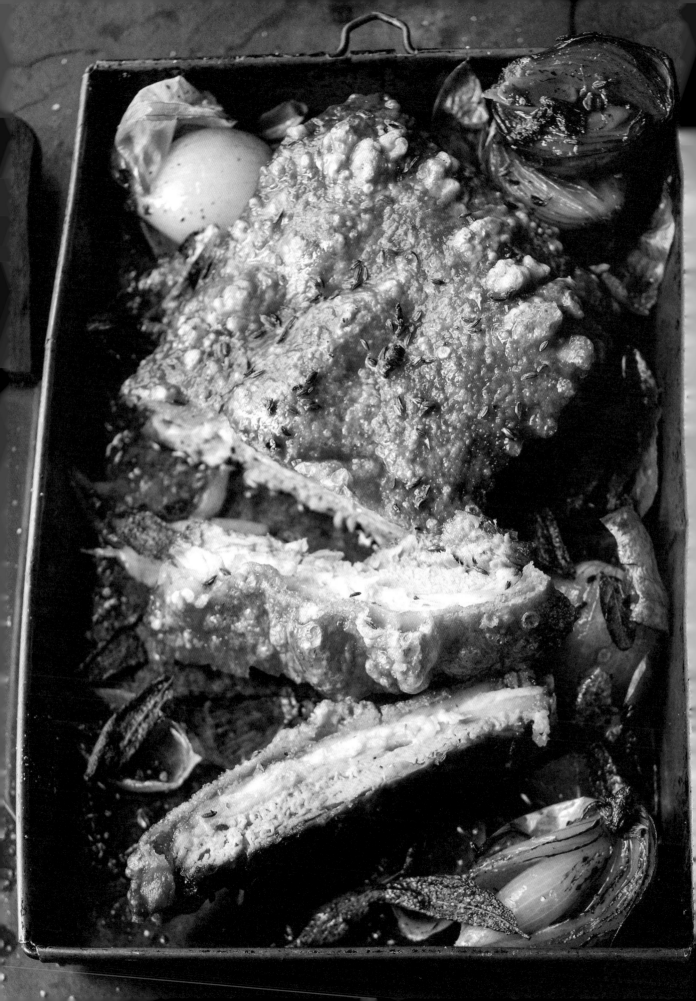

RUBBED LEG OF LAMB WITH CHIMICHURRI

SERVES 4

Argentineans are very aware of the best things to serve with slow cooked lamb. They usually cook whole lambs on massive crosses next to big fires for up to seven hours (it is called Osado), but this recipe is much quicker. We've given you a delicious spice rub for the cooking process and a classic Argentine green sauce called chimichurri to top it with at the end.

3 tbsp coriander seeds

2 tbsp fennel seeds

2 tbsp coarse sea salt

1 tbsp dried thyme

½ tbsp black pepper

¼ tsp cayenne pepper

Splash of coconut oil

1 kg deboned leg of lamb

FOR THE CHIMICHURRI

Large handful fresh parsley, picked and washed

Large handful fresh coriander, picked and washed

Medium handful fresh oregano leaves, picked and washed

4 garlic cloves, crushed

½ red onion, very finely chopped

2 tbsp red wine vinegar (optional)

½ cup extra virgin olive oil

Juice of one fresh lime

Salt and pepper to taste

★ Light the BBQ or preheat the oven to 180°C (Gas 4). (In South Africa we love a braai – or barbecue – and I much prefer doing this on the fire on a gentle heat. The charred flavour you get is incomparable to oven roasting – weather permitting, though.)

★ Combine the coriander, fennel seeds, sea salt, thyme, black pepper and cayenne pepper in a pestle and mortar and pound them roughly. You want some good texture but no whole seeds.

★ Now, add in the coconut oil and mix well, to get a good paste.

★ Massage the paste into the lamb, being sure to cover every bit of it evenly.

★ Either BBQ the meat, turning regularly on a very gentle heat for about 40 minutes, or place in the oven for 40 minutes.

★ Remove the lamb from the heat and rest it for about 10 or 15 minutes. Then, slice finely and serve it with the chimichurri on the side.

★ For the chimichurri, simply chop the herbs as finely as possible, then add them to a bowl along with the garlic, onion, vinegar (if using), oil and lime juice. Mix well with a spoon and season with salt and pepper.

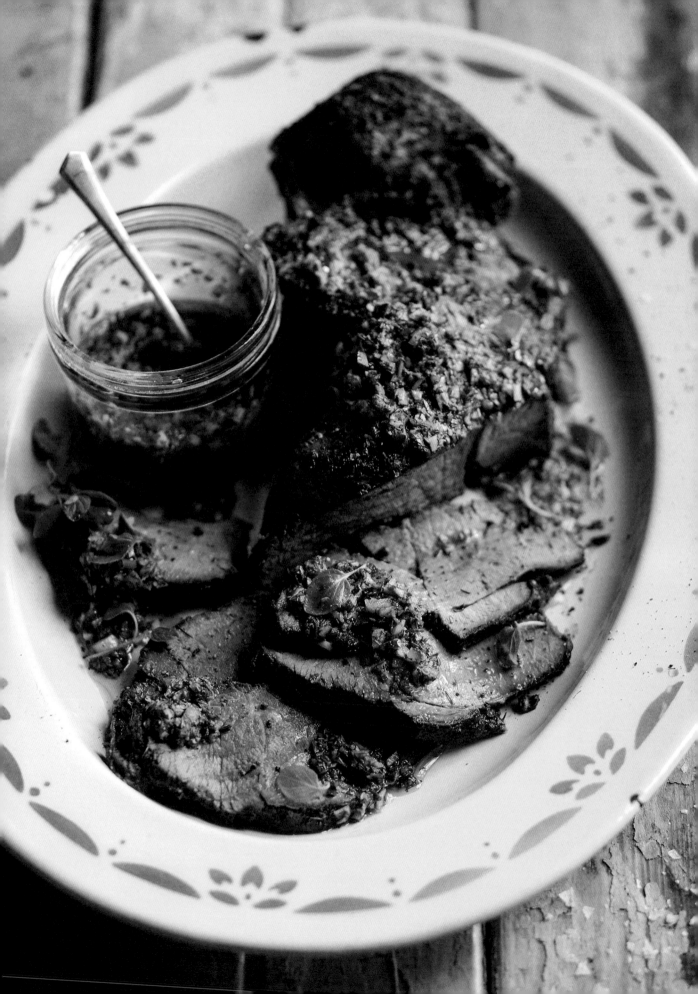

LAMB BLANQUETTE

SERVES 4

This is one of the few stews I make where I don't brown the meat first. I actually don't brown anything off, which is why this is by far the quickest stew one can make. It also happens to be pretty good. The omission of the browning step is what gives this stew the name 'blanquette', which means 'white stew'.

600 g lamb shoulder, cut into 20 g cubes

8 peeled shallots

4 sticks celery, cut into large chunks

5 sprigs thyme

5 sprigs rosemary

2 whole heads garlic, cut in half across the meridian

2 cups chicken stock

1 cup white wine

125 ml cream

2 bunches of leeks, trimmed and cut into big chunks

250 g white or button mushrooms, whole

Salt and pepper

Handful of parsley, freshly chopped

125 ml crème fraîche

★ Preheat the oven to 160°C (Gas 3).

★ Place the lamb, shallots, celery, thyme, rosemary, garlic, stock and wine in an ovenproof casserole dish.

★ Cover the dish with foil and place it in the oven for two and half hours.

★ Check the meat to see whether it is soft and tender. If it is still tough, pop it back in for another 30 minutes.

★ If it is melt-in-the-mouth tender, drain all of the juices from the tray, including the fat, through a sieve into a pot and simmer to reduce.

★ Once all of the liquid has reduced to about 400 ml, add the cream, along with the leek chunks and mushrooms, and reduce the sauce until it goes thick and creamy.

★ Once the sauce is thick and the mushrooms and leeks are tender, add the meat, season with salt and pepper and stir through the freshly chopped parsley.

★ Finally, garnish with dollops of crème fraîche and serve.

Note: If you're splashing out, splash some truffle oil over this before serving. It will be truffle oil well spent. This stew also goes brilliantly with buttered broccoli or 'cauli-rice' (page 70).

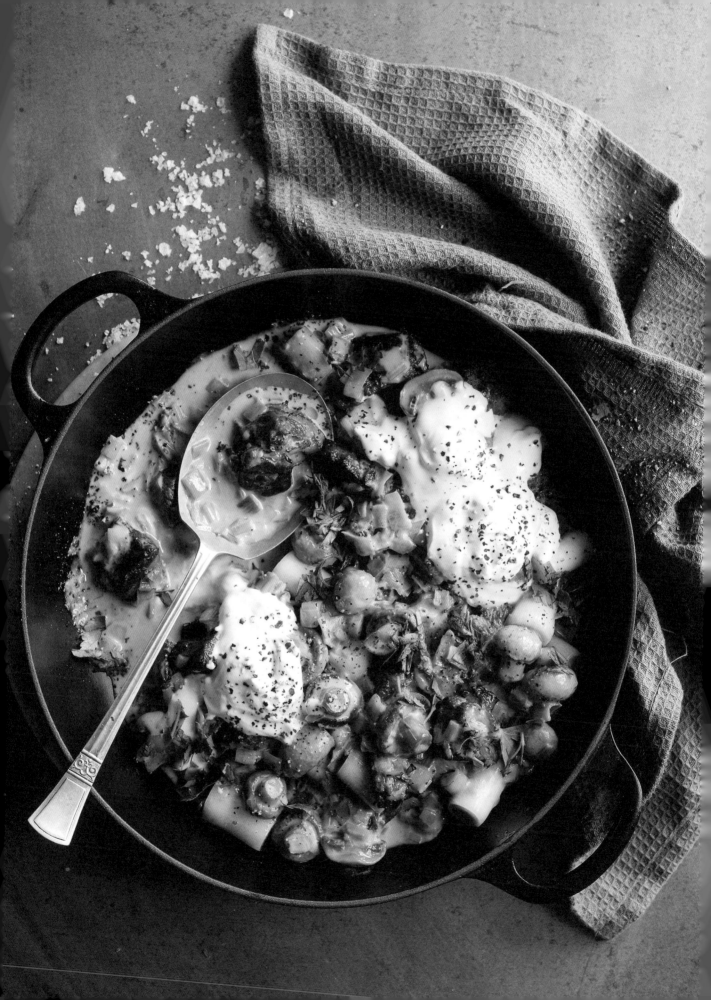

GREEN CURRY PORK STIR-FRY

SERVES 2

1 garlic clove, finely chopped

1 tbsp fish sauce

Juice of 1 lime

½ cup chicken stock

2 tsp Thai green curry paste

200 ml coconut milk

1 handful fresh coriander, finely chopped

1 handful fresh basil leaves, roughly chopped

1 tbsp coconut oil plus extra for frying

350 g pork fillet, thinly sliced

½ cup bean sprouts

80 g mangetouts, julienned

1 red pepper, deseeded and julienned

2 spring onions, finely sliced

★ Combine the garlic, fish sauce, lime juice, chicken stock, curry paste, coconut milk and herbs together in a small bowl and mix well.

★ Heat the oil in a wok and give it a swirl to coat the entire surface.

★ Once the wok reaches a ferocious heat, add the pork and stir-fry for about two minutes or until the meat is cooked – then remove the meat to a separate dish.

★ Place the wok back on the heat and add in a little more coconut oil.

★ Now, add to the wok the bean sprouts, mangetouts, peppers and spring onions and sauté them until they are almost cooked.

★ Add the sauce mixture and boil for two minutes for the flavours to infuse. Then add the pork and warm through.

★ Serve immediately as is or with 'cauli-rice' (page 70).

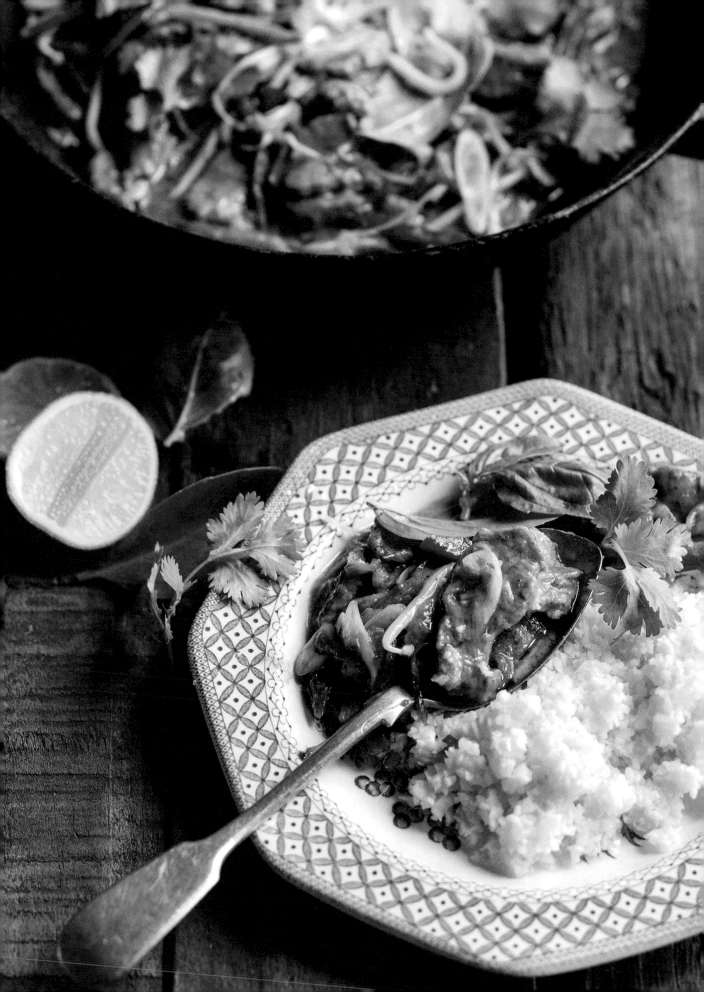

LASAGNE

SERVES 6

If you're not keen on making pasta, use sliced aubergine or courgettes instead.

1 quantity Banting 'pasta' (page 78) or four large aubergines sliced

FOR THE MINCE

250 g streaky bacon

400 g fatty beef mince

40 g butter

2 large onions, finely chopped

2–3 garlic cloves minced

50 g tomato paste

½ cup red wine

1 cup beef stock

3 large sprigs thyme, chopped

1 tin (400 g) chopped tomatoes

1 tbsp Worcestershire sauce

3 large sprigs oregano, chopped

Salt and pepper

FOR THE CHEESE SAUCE

2 cups cream

4 cups grated cheese (Cheddar or Parmesan)

Salt and pepper

1 pinch grated nutmeg

3 egg yolks

Extra cheese for the top

★ In a medium-sized heavy-based frying pan, sauté the bacon and the mince in the butter until golden brown.

★ Once the mince is brown, remove the meat, leaving the fat in the pan. Add the onions to the fat and sauté them until golden brown. Now add the garlic and sauté until aromatic.

★ Return the mince to the pan along with the tomato paste and stir until a dark sediment collects on the base of the pot (this sediment gives the lasagne an amazing roasted flavour).

★ Once a good sediment has collected, add the red wine and reduce it by half while stirring constantly.

★ Now add the beef stock, thyme and the tinned tomatoes and let it simmer on a low heat for about an hour.

★ Add the Worcestershire sauce and oregano and season to taste with salt and pepper.

★ To make the cheese sauce, bring the cream to the boil, then add the cheese, reduce the heat and stir continuously until the cheese has melted and the sauce is a good cheesy consistency.

★ Season with salt, pepper and a pinch of nutmeg then stir in the egg yolks before pouring the sauce over the lasagne.

★ To assemble the lasagne, lay sheets of 'pasta' or sliced aubergine out on the base of a lasagne dish. Cover those sheets with a third of the mince. Cover with another layer of pasta or aubergine, then another layer of mince and another layer of pasta or aubergine. Now top with the final layer of mince, pour over the cheese sauce and sprinkle the grated cheese over.

★ Bake in a preheated oven at 180°C (Gas 4) for 30 to 45 minutes.

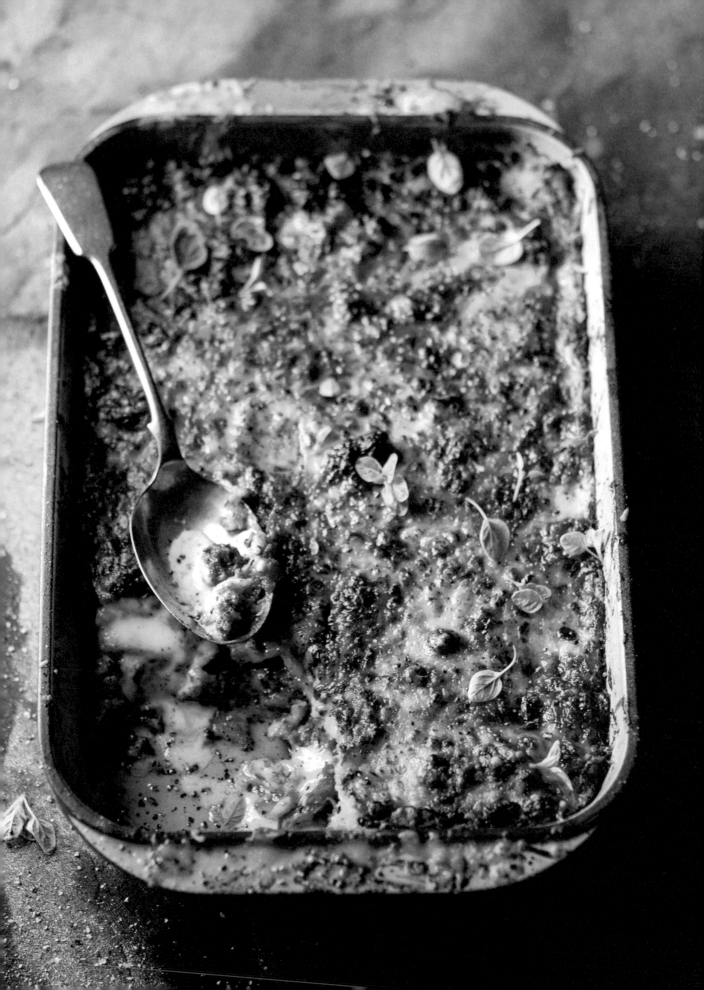

SMOKY PORK BROTH

SERVES 2

If you haven't thrown your smoky pork hock into your mother's special pea and ham soup, we strongly recommend using it for a rich pork broth. Broths are so rarely made using pork bones but the pig has some of the best flavour you can get. You can use smoked or un-smoked bones for your broth; it depends entirely on your palate.

½ red onion, sliced

1 red pepper, deseeded and sliced

100 g gammon steak, cut into chunks

1 tbsp butter

1 garlic clove, crushed

500 ml smoky pork stock (or other stock – see basic broth recipe on page 64)

2 pieces orange zest

80 g sugar snap peas cut in half on the angle

½ cup cherry tomatoes

½ tsp smoked paprika

Juice of 1 lemon

2 large sprigs oregano, washed and picked

Salt and pepper

★ In a medium-sized saucepan, sauté the onion, peppers and gammon in butter until they begin to caramelize.

★ Add the garlic and sauté until aromatic.

★ Now, add the broth and the orange zest and bring to the boil for 5 minutes.

★ Then add the sugar snap peas, cherry tomatoes, smoked paprika and lemon juice and simmer for 5 minutes.

★ Finally, add the oregano and season to taste with salt and pepper.

Note: This soup does well with anything smoky or porky added. If you have bacon, pork belly, sausages or even black pudding, chuck them in.

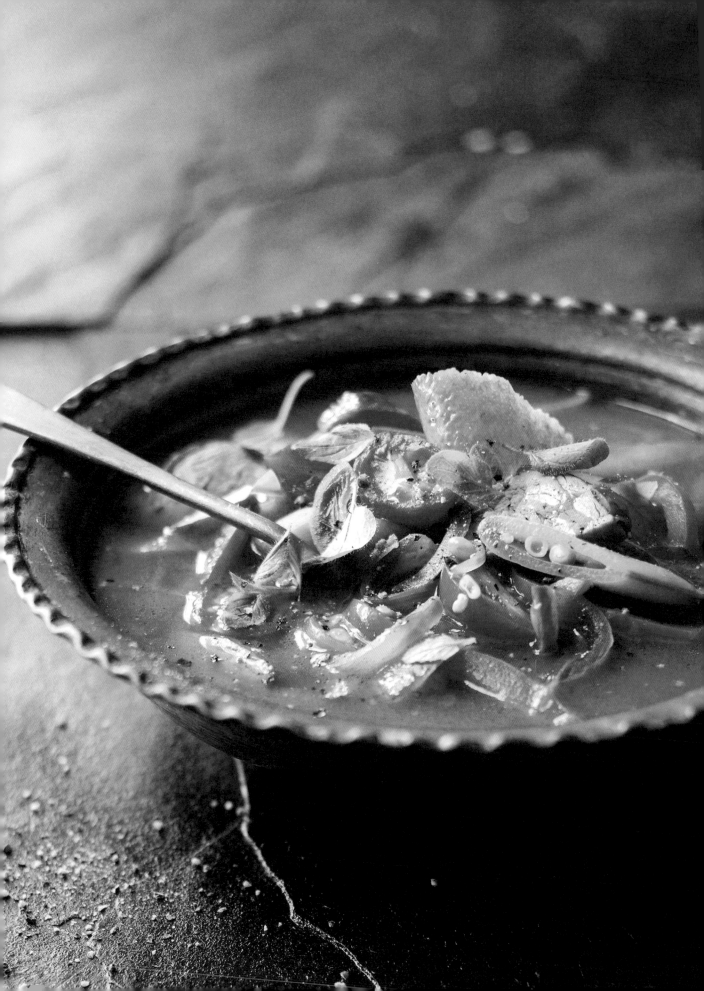

CARPACCIO WITH PARMESAN AND CAPERS

SERVES 4

If you're entertaining, carpaccio is a perfect dish to prep in advance. Simply follow the steps, slice it onto a platter and keep it covered in the fridge until service time.

Salt and pepper

A few sprigs thyme, finely chopped

500 g beef fillet

1 tbsp coconut oil

FOR THE MARINADE

½ red onion, sliced

3 tbsp chopped parsley

1 tsp Dijon mustard

Juice of half a lemon

4 tbsp olive oil

2 tbsp chopped capers

GARNISH

100 g Parmesan shavings

Large handful wild rocket leaves

★ Season the beef with lots of salt and pepper and rub the thyme over the meat.

★ Heat a heavy-based pan on the stove with a little coconut oil and sear the beef in the pan for no longer than a minute, just until it has colour all around it. Remove from the pan.

★ Slice the fillet as thinly as you can with a sharp knife.

★ Place each slice on your chopping board and flatten with the flat side of your knife, then lay each slice on a platter.

★ Mix together all the ingredients for the marinade in a bowl. Drizzle the marinade over the meat and season well with salt and pepper.

★ Garnish the dish by scattering with Parmesan shavings and wild rocket.

Note: You can swap the beef fillet in the recipe for fresh tuna.

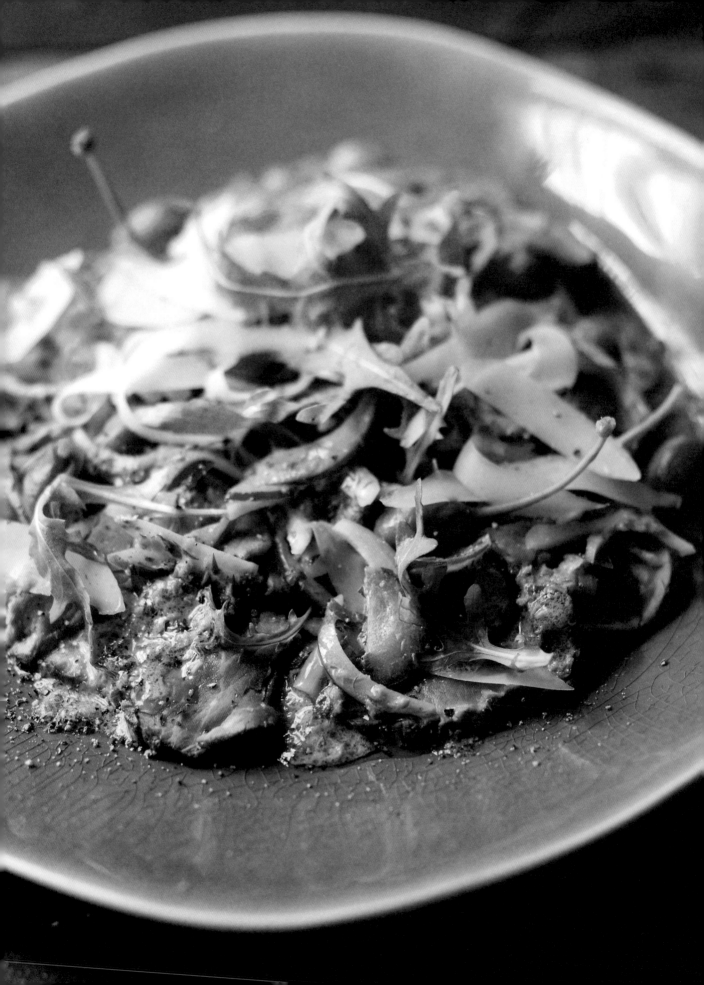

LAMB KOFTA WITH TZATZIKI

SERVES 4

Kofta is a classic North African dish, although a few countries in the Middle East, along with Greece and Turkey, will claim these meatballs as theirs. To avoid offending anyone, you're welcome to call the tzatziki 'cucumber yoghurt'.

FOR THE KOFTA

Coconut oil or ghee for frying

1 onion, chopped

2 garlic cloves, crushed

1 tsp salt

1 tbsp ground coriander

1 tsp ground cumin

½ tsp ground cinnamon

½ tsp ground allspice

¼ tsp cayenne pepper

¼ tsp ground ginger

1 handful flat-leaf parsley, roughly chopped

800 g lamb mince

Salt and black pepper

FOR THE TZATZIKI

½ cucumber, halved and seeded

Salt

½ garlic clove

1 tbsp olive oil

1 tbsp lemon juice

½ tbsp fresh mint, finely chopped

1 cup double thick Greek yoghurt

★ Sauté the onions and garlic in oil until softened.

★ Add the spices to the pan and sauté them with the onions until they become aromatic.

★ Mix the pan contents, the chopped parsley and the mince together in a bowl and season well.

★ Divide the meat mixture into about 12 rough balls.

★ Mould each piece around the pointed end of a bamboo kebab skewer. They should look little lamb rugby balls (or American footballs) on the end of the skewers. Cover and refrigerate for at least 1 hour before grilling.

★ Heat a griddle pan or frying pan over some serious heat, or prepare a BBQ grill.

★ Brush the meat lightly with some melted coconut oil or ghee, then place them in the pan or on the grill.

★ Give them about three minutes on each side to allow them to colour properly, then serve with tzatziki.

★ To make the tzatziki, grate the cucumber and place in a strainer. Sprinkle it with salt and mix with your hands or a spoon. Then leave it to strain for about half an hour. Wring the moisture out of the cucumber using your hands, then stir the cucumber, garlic, olive oil, lemon juice and mint into the yoghurt. Refrigerate for at least 1 hour before serving.

Note: When using wooden skewers be sure to soak them in water for at least 15 minutes before using them.

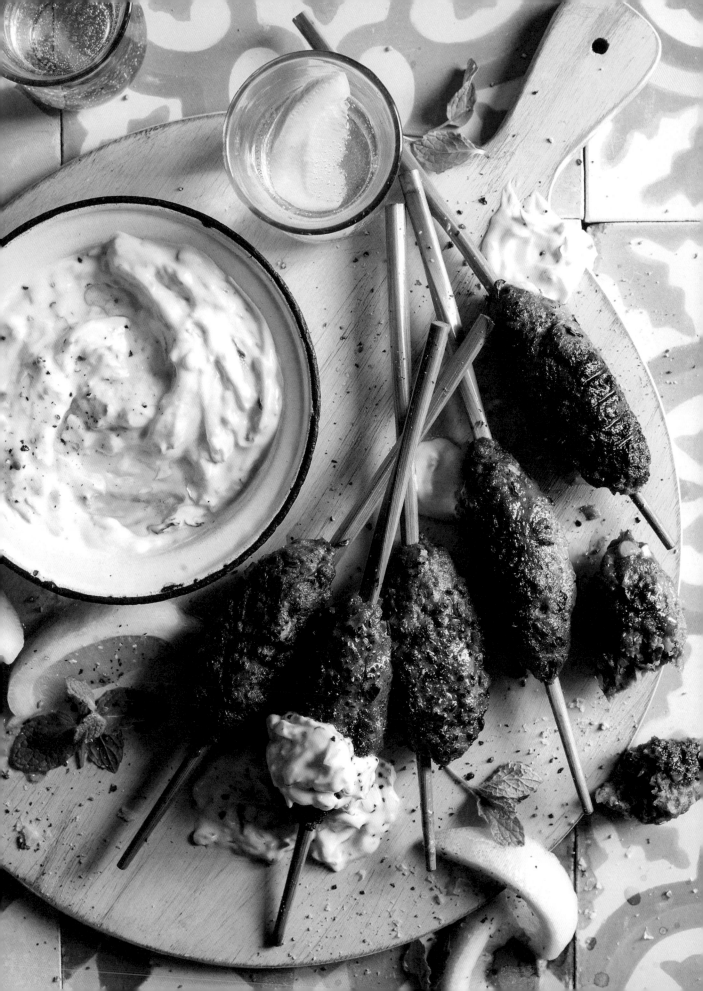

BANGERS AND MASH

SERVES 4

With Britain embracing Banting, one might imagine a national shift away from one of the country's most famous dishes. In this recipe we've made use of cauli-mash to save the Brits and the rest of the Western world from a life without bangers and mash.

50 g butter

8 pork sausages
(100 per cent pork)

100 g bacon, diced

2 red onions, sliced

4 garlic cloves, peeled and crushed

4 sprigs rosemary

500 g plum tomatoes, quartered

1 cup chicken stock

★ Preheat the oven to 200°C (Gas 6).

★ Melt the butter in a pan and sear the sausages, then set aside.

★ Fry the bacon in the pan until crispy then add the onions, garlic and rosemary and fry until the onion is softened.

★ Add the tomatoes and cook for about 10 minutes until the tomatoes start breaking down.

★ Add the chicken stock, pour everything into a baking tray and place the sausages on top.

★ Bake in the oven for 20 minutes.

★ Serve with buttery 'cauli-mash' (see recipe on page 68).

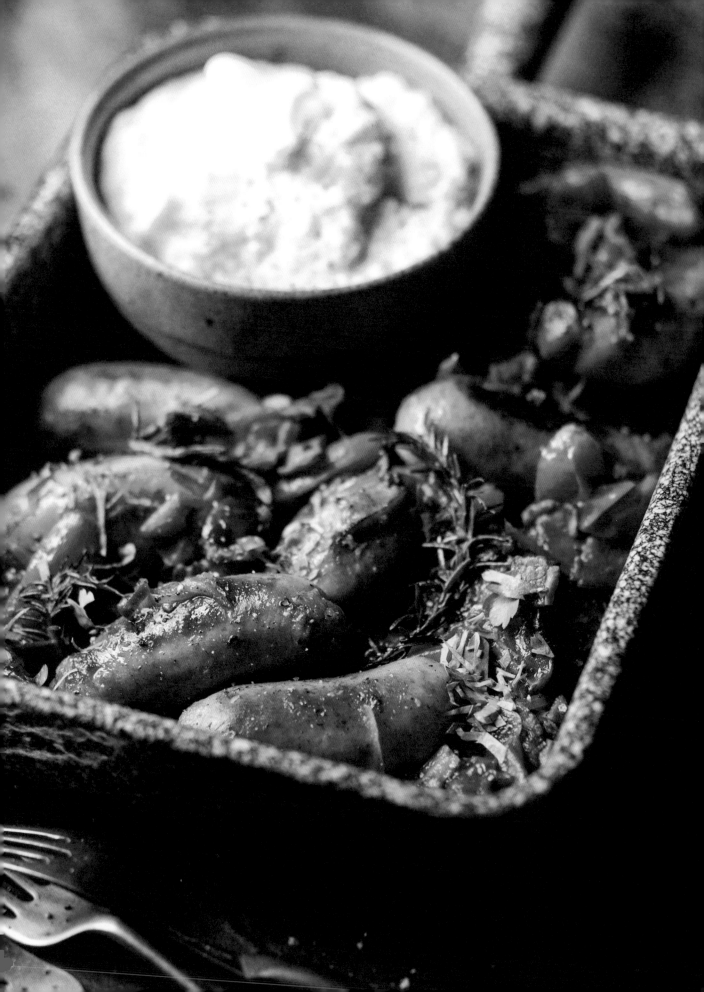

GAMMON AND MUSTARD CABBAGE ROLLS

MAKES 4

These cabbage rolls are the easiest alternative to standard tortilla wraps. A total winner!

4 large cabbage leaves

½ cup mayonnaise

1 pickled onion, halved and sliced

1 large pickled cucumber, diced

½ red onion, finely diced

1 tbsp capers, rinsed and chopped

1 tbsp chopped parsley

1 tbsp Dijon mustard

Squeeze of lemon juice

2 cups shredded white cabbage

½ cup pecan nuts, toasted and chopped

2 boiled eggs, roughly chopped

50 g crispy bacon pieces

8 slices good-quality ham

★ Blanch the cabbage leaves in boiling salted water until they are soft and refresh by plunging them into cold water.

★ Mix all of the remaining ingredients together, apart from the blanched leaves and the gammon.

★ Lay each blanched cabbage leaf flat and place two pieces of ham on each one.

★ Fill each leaf with the coleslaw mixture, then roll them like spring rolls or burritos.

★ Slice the wraps once through the middle and serve with some mayonnaise and mustard.

Note: You can fill these cabbage wraps with absolutely anything. We just like the cabbage slaw because you get great mileage out of one cabbage.

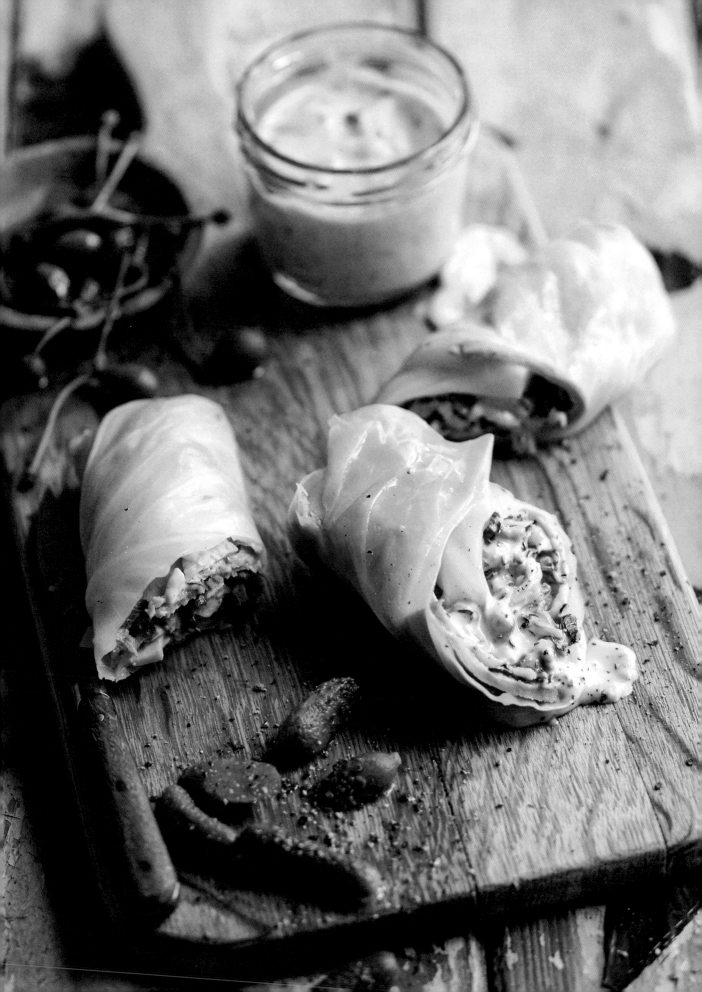

POULTRY

In many parts of the world, the variety of poultry available is becoming increasingly limited. Turkeys only really come around once a year and ducks are expensive. One of the reasons is the fact that chickens are manufactured at such an alarming rate that hardly anything else can compete on price. As you will have read earlier in this book, we are completely against this kind of farming. When you use chicken, duck or turkey in any of the recipes that follow, we urge you to choose the organic ones. All 'free-range' means is that they're not in cages, but they still walk around in massive barns and are often raised on questionable feed.

On a lighter note, organic chickens are still cheaper than most other meats.

Chermoula chicken kebabs

Not-butter chicken

Creamy butter chicken curry

Parmesan chicken pieces with roast garlic tomato mole

Chicken livers peri-peri

Roast chicken

Crispy roasted duck

Kung pao chicken on coconut 'cauli-rice'

Creamy simmered chicken with olives, salami and capers

Ponzu duck salad with cucumber noodles

Chicken and coconut broth

Spicy chicken wings with blue cheese dip

CHERMOULA CHICKEN KEBABS

SERVES 4

Chermoula is a brilliant Moroccan marinade that is traditionally used on lamb. We've given you a chermoula recipe that we use but if you don't have that kind of time, an organic pre-packed variety could save you half an hour. Serve with dukkah yoghurt.

FOR THE CHICKEN KEBABS

8 large bamboo skewers, soaked in water

2 yellow peppers, deseeded and cut into squares

16 deboned chicken thighs, each cut into three

FOR THE CHERMOULA

1½ tbsp ground coriander

2 tbsp ground cumin

1 heaped tbsp turmeric

½ tsp dried red chilli

½ tsp coarse salt

3 tsp paprika

1 garlic clove, minced

1 tbsp tomato paste

1 handful fresh parsley

1 handful fresh coriander

Juice of two lemons

1 cup olive oil

FOR THE DUKKAH YOGHURT

1 cup thick Greek yoghurt

1 garlic clove, mashed

2 tbsp dry dukkah

Salt and pepper

★ First, make the yoghurt. Combine all of the ingredients and leave to stand for an hour to infuse.

★ Then, make the chermoula (if you've bought chermoula, skip this step). Purée all of the ingredients into a fine paste, then turn out into a saucepan and cook for about 15 minutes until the oil begins to split from the mixture. Store in a sterilized jar for up to a month in the fridge.

★ Make the kebabs by skewering a square of pepper followed by a piece of chicken and continue the pattern until you have six pieces of chicken on each skewer.

★ Pour the chermoula over the chicken and rub it in.

★ You can grill the kebabs straight away but leaving them for a while, or even overnight, will enhance the flavour dramatically.

★ Cook them on as high a temperature as possible until nice and dark on the outside and serve with the dukkah yoghurt on the side.

Note: Fresh coriander and a twist of fresh lime are a perfect garnish to freshen this dish up.

Dukkah is a North African spice and nut mix available in many delis and supermarkets.

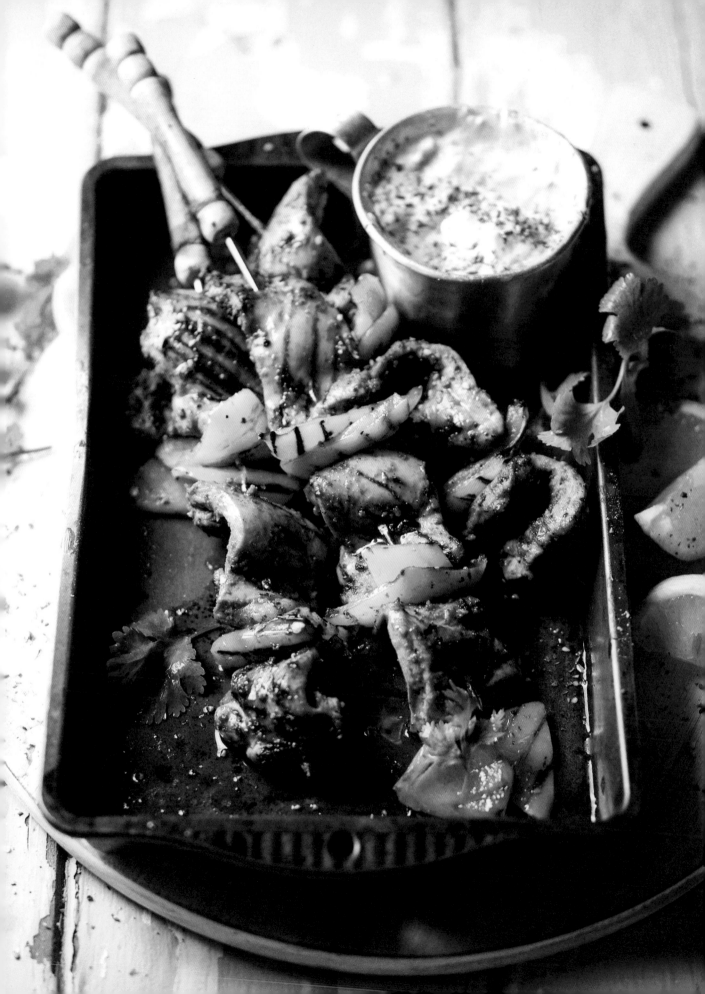

NOT-BUTTER CHICKEN

SERVES 6

As the name might suggest, this is not a traditional butter chicken curry. Having said that, it is a much more appropriate interpretation for the term 'butter chicken', as it is literally chicken cooked in butter. It also tastes like butter, which makes it more like butter chicken than butter chicken could ever be. But still, it's definitely not butter chicken.

1 onion, sliced

250 g button mushrooms, cut into quarters

4 sprigs thyme

1 whole head of garlic, cut in half down the middle

6 chicken legs

1 cup chicken stock

1 cup double cream

1 cup white wine

120 g butter, broken into 6 little knobs

Salt and pepper

★ Preheat the oven to 160°C (Gas 3).

★ Place the onions, mushrooms, thyme sprigs and the garlic head in an oven-proof tray, spreading them out evenly.

★ Press the chicken legs skin side up on top of the vegetables. The tray should be tightly packed and have as little space as possible between the pieces of chicken.

★ Now, cover the chicken with the stock, cream and wine.

★ Place a knob of butter on top of each chicken piece and bake in the oven, uncovered, for 1 hour and 30 minutes.

★ Strain the sauce off into a saucepan and reduce it by a third by simmering gently. Pour this back over the chicken and reheat in the oven before serving.

Note: The sauce is perfect with 'cauli-rice' or 'cauli-mash' (see page 68).

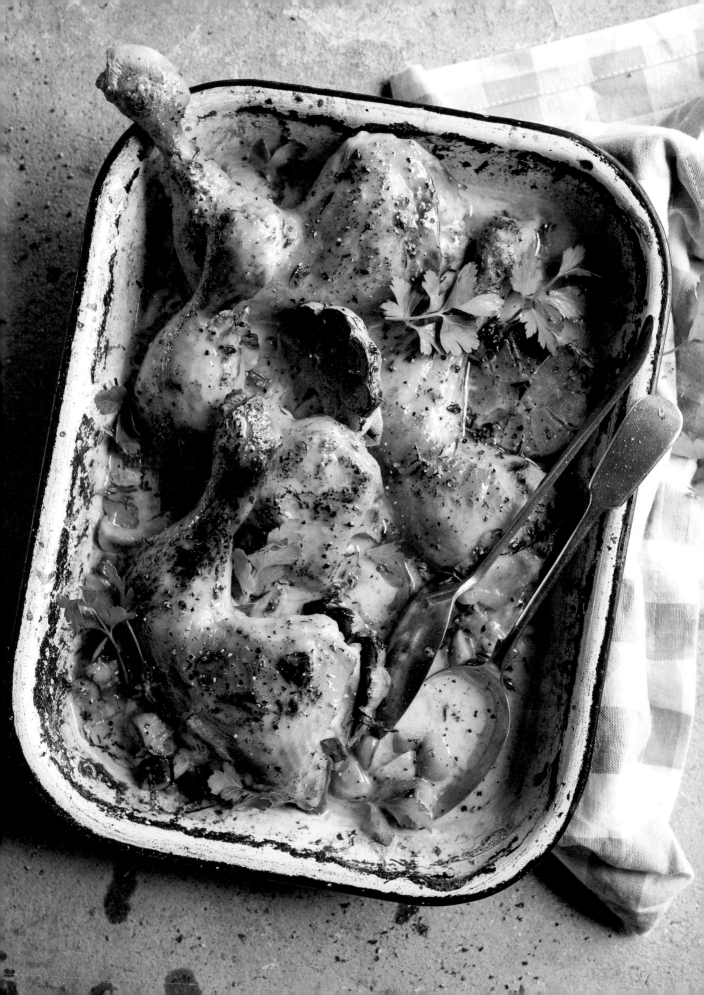

CREAMY BUTTER CHICKEN CURRY

SERVES 8

If you'll excuse the irony, the previous 'butter chicken' recipe might not have been a traditional butter chicken curry, but this one definitely is. A great way to indulge in a takeaway favourite – but much healthier.

FOR THE CHICKEN
½ cup plain yoghurt

1 tbsp ground cumin

1 tbsp ground coriander

1 tsp ground turmeric

1 knob ginger, grated

2 garlic cloves, minced

8 chicken breasts, cut into large cubes

Butter for frying

FOR THE SAUCE
4 tbsp butter

4 garlic cloves, minced

2 knobs ginger, grated

1 tbsp ground cumin

1 tbsp ground coriander

½ tsp paprika

½ tsp cayenne pepper

400 g tomato purée or passata

1 cup double cream

180 ml coconut milk

1 tsp garam masala

Salt and pepper to taste

1 handful fresh curry leaves

1 handful fresh coriander, roughly chopped for garnish

★ Preheat the oven to 200°C (Gas 6).

★ Combine all of the ingredients for the marinade and smear the mixture over the chicken. Leave to stand for 30 minutes or so.

★ While the chicken is marinating, make the sauce. Melt the butter in a saucepan, then add the garlic and ginger and sauté for a minute or so. Now, add the spices and let them toast for a minute. Add the tomato purée or passata and let it cook down by half. When the tomato has thickened and is no longer acidic, add the cream and coconut milk and allow it to simmer and reduce until it has slightly thickened. Add the garam masala and the curry leaves and season to taste with salt and pepper.

★ Heat a frying pan with a little butter and sear the chicken cubes. Try to put colour on the chicken, but not cook it through.

★ Finally, add the chicken to the simmering sauce and cook for about five minutes. Garnish with chopped coriander.

Note: Serve this with your favourite sambals, a tomato and onion salad, and cucumber yoghurt. We often use some of our amazing cauli-wraps (page 82) as naan replacements too.

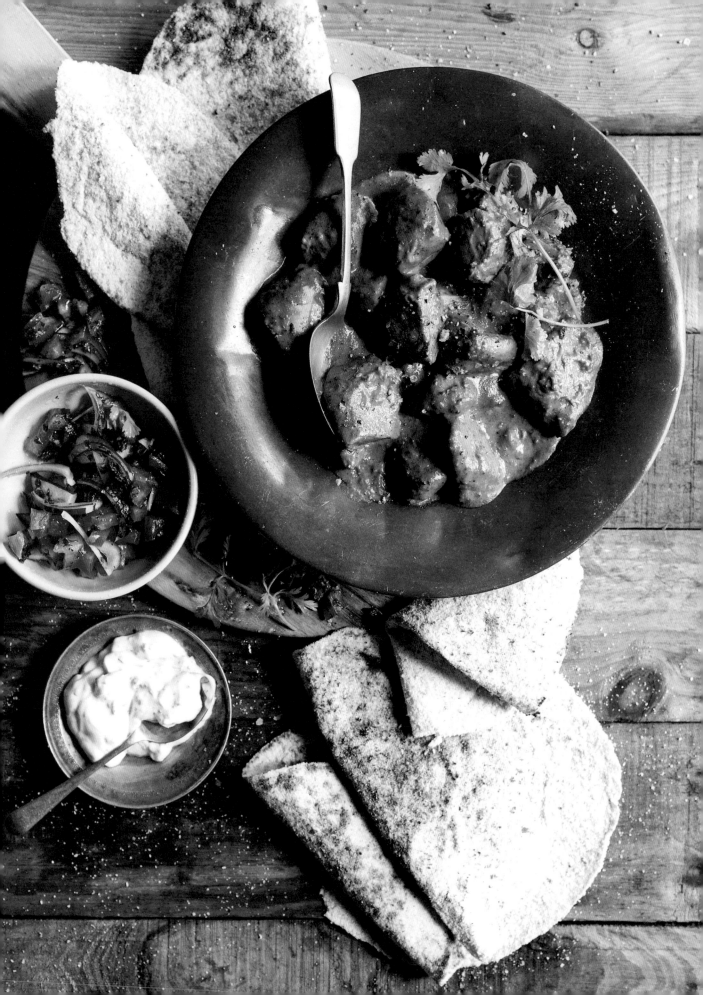

PARMESAN CHICKEN PIECES WITH ROAST GARLIC TOMATO MOLE

SERVES 4

Parmesan crumbing is a great technique to take the place of bread crumbing. In this recipe we add in a Spanish twist with the smoky mole sauce.

FOR THE MOLE SAUCE

1 whole head garlic

60 g butter

1 onion, roughly chopped

1 tin (400 g) whole peeled tomatoes

1 tbsp sweet smoked paprika

1 handful fresh oregano, roughly chopped

Salt and pepper

FOR THE CHICKEN

½ cup finely grated Parmesan cheese

¼ cup almond flour

Salt and pepper

4 medium-sized chicken breasts

1 egg, beaten

50 g butter

Note: For a zing of acidity, you could add a squeeze of lemon to the mole sauce.

★ Preheat the oven to 180°C (Gas 4).

★ Slice the top from the garlic and press half the butter into the meat of it. Wrap in tinfoil and leave it, upright, in the oven for 45 minutes.

★ Meanwhile, fry the onions on a low heat in a small pot in the rest of the butter. Once they turn golden brown, add the tinned tomatoes and smoked paprika.

★ Cook this on a low heat for about ten minutes. If it goes too dry, add a drop or two of water.

★ When the time is up, remove the garlic from the oven and squeeze the flesh straight into the sauce. Add the oregano and give a last minute or two of heat.

★ Using a potato masher, mash the tomatoes and the garlic together to form a thick, chunky, smoky tomato sauce. Season with salt and pepper.

★ Mix the Parmesan and almond flour together, season with salt and pepper and spread the mixture out on a plate or tray.

★ Wet the chicken breasts by dunking them into the beaten egg. Then drop them into the Parmesan and almond mix, making sure there is an even coating on each side.

★ Melt the butter on a medium heat in a heavy-based frying pan and grill each chicken breast on both sides until golden brown.

★ If they are not completely cooked through (check by cutting into them with a knife, the juices should run clear), finish off in the oven (this also helps prevent the crumbs from burning or falling apart). In total they should cook for about ten minutes.

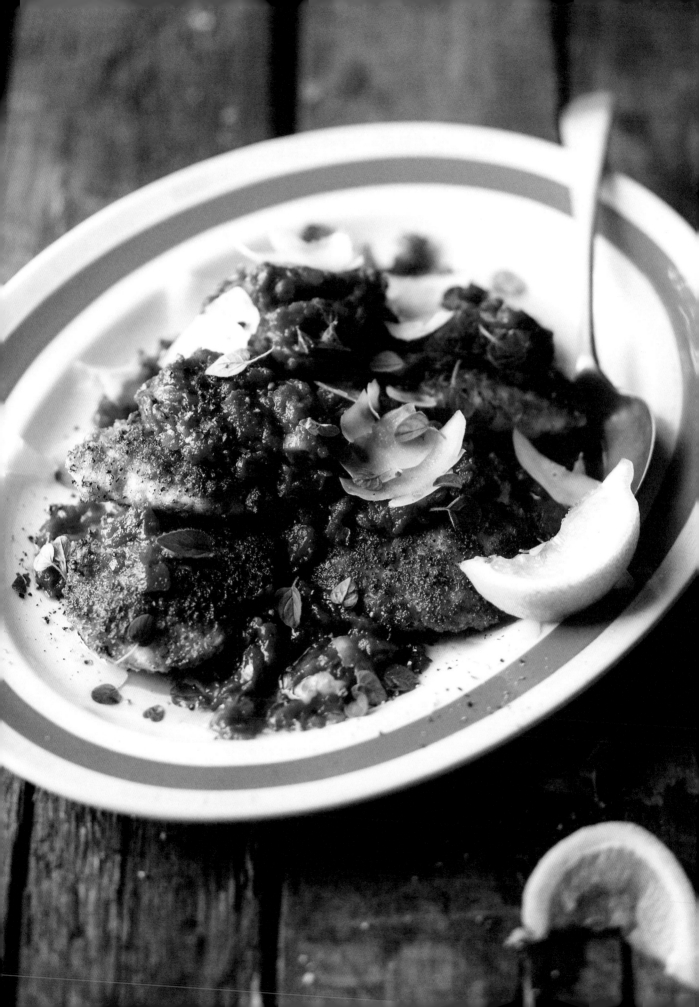

CHICKEN LIVERS PERI-PERI

SERVES 2

The secret to great livers is to cook them in a fiercely hot pan. Here, the ingredients are very simple but following the steps in the right order is paramount!

Butter for frying

1 large onion, sliced

4 garlic cloves, roughly chopped

2 red chillies, deseeded and chopped

½ cup white wine

1 cup tomato purée

1 large lemon, juiced

Salt and pepper

250 g chicken livers

Coconut oil for frying

1 handful basil, roughly chopped

★ Make the sauce first by sautéing the onions in butter on a low heat until they are soft, sweet and golden brown. Add the garlic and chillies and sauté until fragrant, then add the wine and reduce by half. Then add the tomato purée and the lemon juice and simmer for a minute. Season to taste with salt and pepper and set aside.

★ Clean the livers of their gallbladders (the green bit that looks like a dill pickle) and then cut them into bite-size pieces.

★ Pat each liver dry with paper towel. This helps prevent the livers from boiling in their own juices. Now, season them with salt and pepper.

★ Get a large heavy-based frying pan smoking hot, then add in a tiny bit of coconut oil.

★ Drop the livers in and spread them quickly so there are none sitting on top of each other. It will be hot, so be careful.

★ Turn each piece using a fork or spatula but DO NOT stir them. You want to keep them as still as possible in the pan so they get great colour and do not leach their juices.

★ When they are nice and brown on each side, pour the sauce back into the pan and simmer for a minute or two.

★ Season with salt and pepper and sprinkle with the fresh basil. Check the seasoning one last time and serve immediately.

Note: It sucks eating chicken livers without soft, floury bread, but give it a bash on some of our cauliflower mash (page 68). You won't be disappointed!

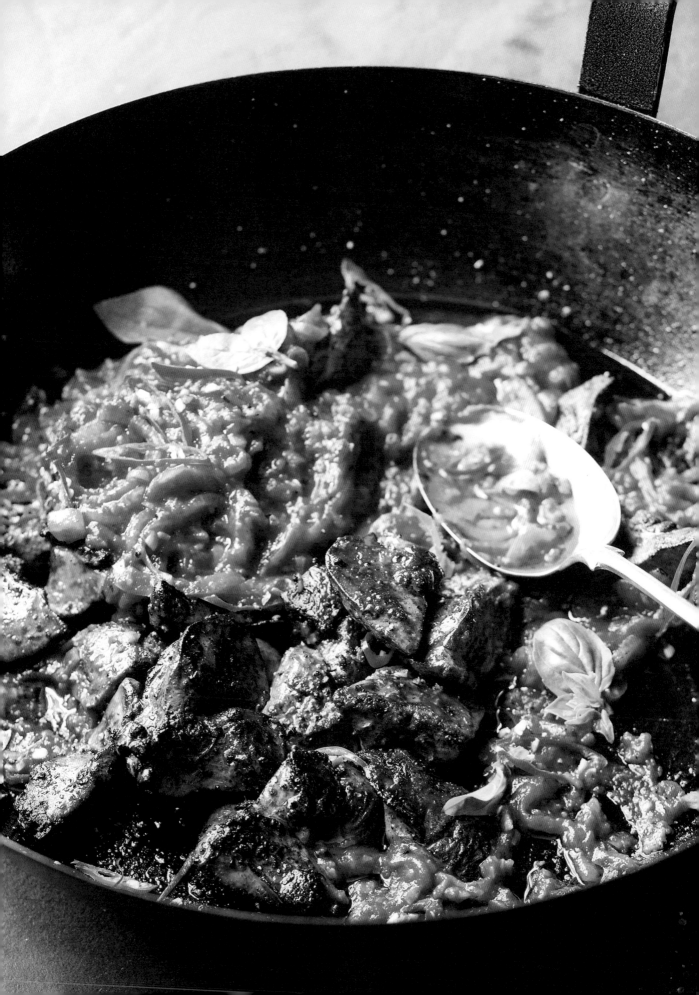

ROAST CHICKEN

SERVES 4

The roast chicken is a Banting staple. If you roast it properly, not only do you get some good fat in the tray for later use, and obviously heaps of protein, but more importantly, once you've finished carving you can bang that carcass straight into water to make a broth as you saw in the 'basics' section on page 64.

1 whole head garlic

1 tbsp dried thyme

1 tbsp dried parsley

1 tbsp dried oregano

4 tbsp melted butter

Salt and pepper

1 white onion, quartered

1 whole chicken

2 lemons, quartered

1 handful fresh thyme leaves

2 red onions, quartered

★ Preheat your oven to 200°C (Gas 6).

★ Slice the garlic in half vertically through the middle.

★ Peel the cloves from one half of the garlic and place them in a pestle and mortar with the herbs and the melted butter.

★ Mash together with some seasoning to make a paste.

★ Rub the chicken all over with the paste and season well with salt and pepper.

★ Place the quarters of one white onion and a lemon in the cavity of the chicken with some of the thyme.

★ Place the remaining ingredients in a roasting tray and add the chicken on top.

★ With a piece of string, tie the legs together to keep the aromatics in the cavity (the most basic form of trussing) .

★ Roast for 1 hour 10 to 1 hour 25 minutes, depending on the size of your chicken. Check to see if the chicken is cooked by placing a skewer in the thickest part of the leg – the juices should run clear. If not, return it to the oven for another 10 minutes and check again.

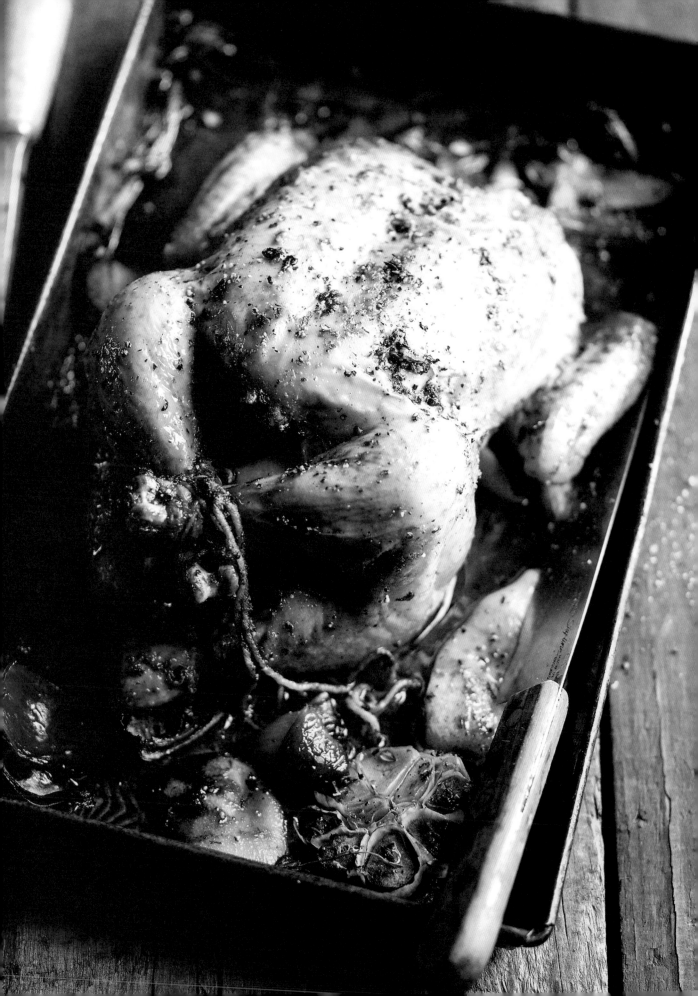

CRISPY ROASTED DUCK

SERVES 4–6

There are hundreds of methods for duck roasting. What I found while testing duck recipes is that they are either crispy, but require a lengthy blanching and drying method, or they are really simple but do not end up going crispy.

This particular recipe is both simple and ends up crispy and delicious. We've served it with our coconut crêpes (page 80), some sliced cucumber and spring onion.

FOR THE DUCK

1 duck (2 kg), innards set aside for the jus

Salt and pepper

1 tbsp fennel seeds

1 cinnamon stick

5 star anise

1 orange, cut into quarters

FOR THE COMPÔTE

300 g frozen or fresh cranberries, roughly chopped

3 tbsp xylitol

★ Preheat the oven to 150°C (Gas 2).

★ Remove the innards from the duck. They come in a bag like chicken giblets, but a butcher would do this for you too. Pat the whole duck dry with paper towel.

★ Using a skewer or a sharp fork, prick holes in the fat over the entire bird.

★ Rub the duck skin with salt and pepper. Place the spices and the orange quarters into the cavity of the duck.

★ Set the duck on a rack in a roasting tray and place it in the oven for four hours. You must take the duck out every hour and turn it.

★ At the end of the cooking time, remove the duck from the oven and crank up the heat to 200°C (Gas 6). Place the duck back in the oven for 10 minutes to let it crisp up.

★ Leave it to rest for 15 minutes, then carve it up and serve.

★ Meanwhile, warm the cranberries in a small saucepan on a gentle heat.

★ Once they release their juices, add the xylitol and let them simmer gently for about ten minutes or until slightly softened.

★ Remove from the heat, allow to cool and purée with a stick blender.

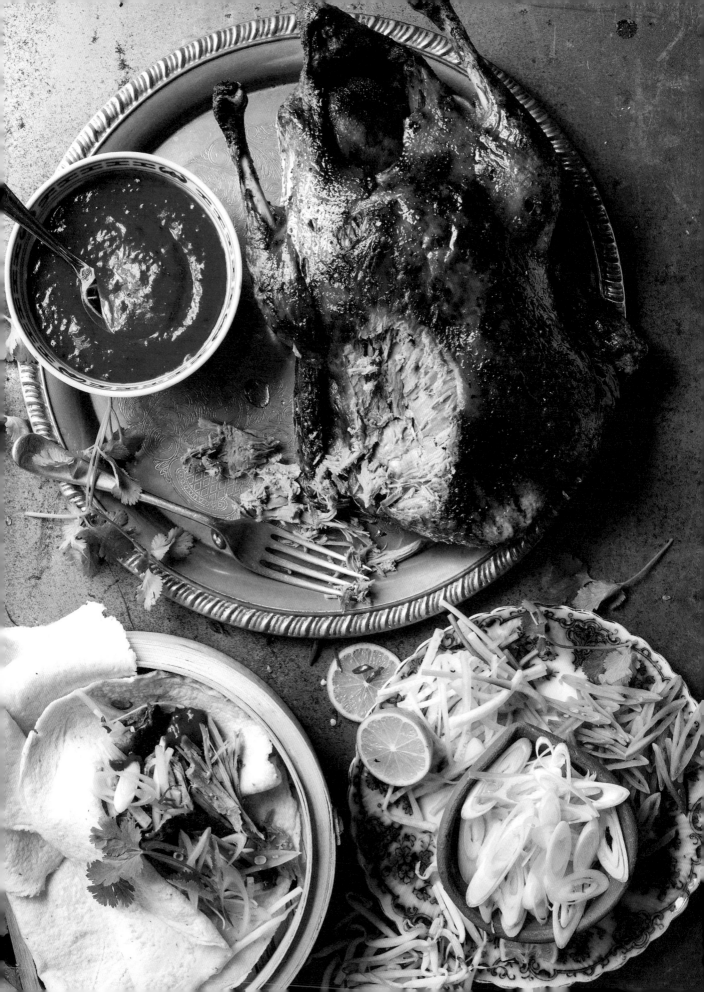

KUNG PAO CHICKEN ON COCONUT 'CAULI-RICE'

SERVES 2

In most cases with chicken, I try to use the thighs. They are much juicier and far more flavoursome, but chicken breasts would work as well. We have given you a basic recipe for 'cauli-rice' in the Banting toolkit at the beginning of the book (see page 70) but this is a nice Asian adaptation.

FOR THE CHICKEN

2 tsp tamari soy sauce (naturally fermented)

2 tsp Chinese rice wine or dry sherry

1 tsp sesame oil

2 tbsp oyster sauce

1 tsp chilli and garlic paste

2 spring onions, finely sliced

1 tsp Szechuan peppercorns (optional)

A few drops sesame oil for frying

400 g boneless, skinless chicken thighs, cut into bite-size pieces

4 tbsp roughly chopped macadamia nuts

FOR THE 'CAULI-RICE'

½ tin (200 ml) coconut milk

½ large cauliflower, cut into chunks

Water

Fish sauce

★ Make the cauli-rice. In a small saucepan, reduce the coconut milk to one third of its original volume on a medium heat.

★ Place the cauliflower in the bowl of a food processor and pulse until it reaches rice consistency.

★ Now, add the cauli-rice to the coconut milk and add enough water to cover the mixture. Stir continuously until the 'rice' is al dente.

★ Season with a splash of fish sauce before serving.

★ Combine the tamari, rice wine, 1 tbsp sesame oil, oyster sauce, chilli and garlic paste, spring onions and peppercorns, if using, in a bowl.

★ Get a wok smoking hot and add a few drops of sesame oil. Seal the chicken off on a high heat until it has good colour and is cooked through.

★ Now, pour the sauce ingredients into the pan and cook until they are boiling.

★ Finally, add the nuts, toss them through and serve the chicken on a bed of steaming coconut cauli-rice.

Note: If you wanted to add some more love to your 'cauli-rice', you could run through some chopped spring onions and coriander.

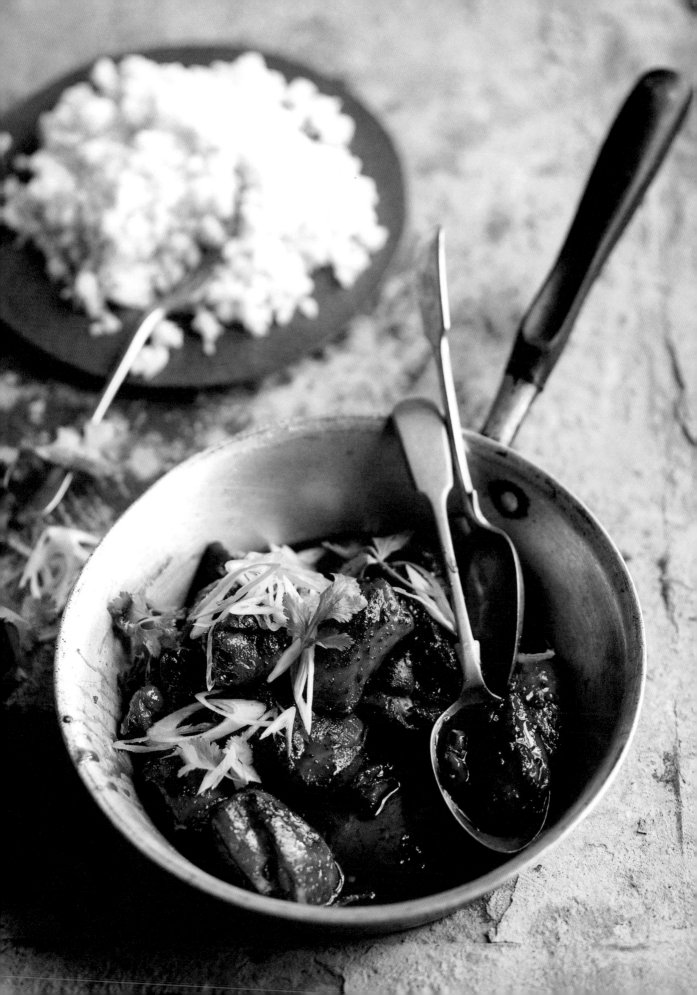

CREAMY SIMMERED CHICKEN WITH OLIVES, SALAMI AND CAPERS

SERVES 2

Simmered chicken breaks the normal rules of sealing the meat, then cooking the vegetables in the same pan for the flavour, then adding the meat back in later. For this recipe, you literally just drop the meat into the boiling sauce and that's it.

80 g butter

1 red onion, sliced

1 red pepper, deseeded and sliced

10 thick slices salami, cut into quarters

2 chicken breasts, skinned (don't throw the skin away) and cut into thin strips

2 tbsp capers

¼ cup green olives

1 cup stock

1 cup double cream

Salt and pepper

★ In a large, heavy-based pan, sauté the onion, pepper, salami and chicken skin in the butter until lightly browned.

★ Then add the capers, olives and the stock and boil until the stock reduces by half.

★ Now add the cream and reduce by a third.

★ Finally, drop the chicken pieces into the sauce and simmer for two or three minutes.

★ Season with salt and pepper and serve.

Note: You can make the exact same recipe but swap the cream for good-quality tomatoes (tinned or fresh). It's very similar to a dish called Chicken Chasseur.

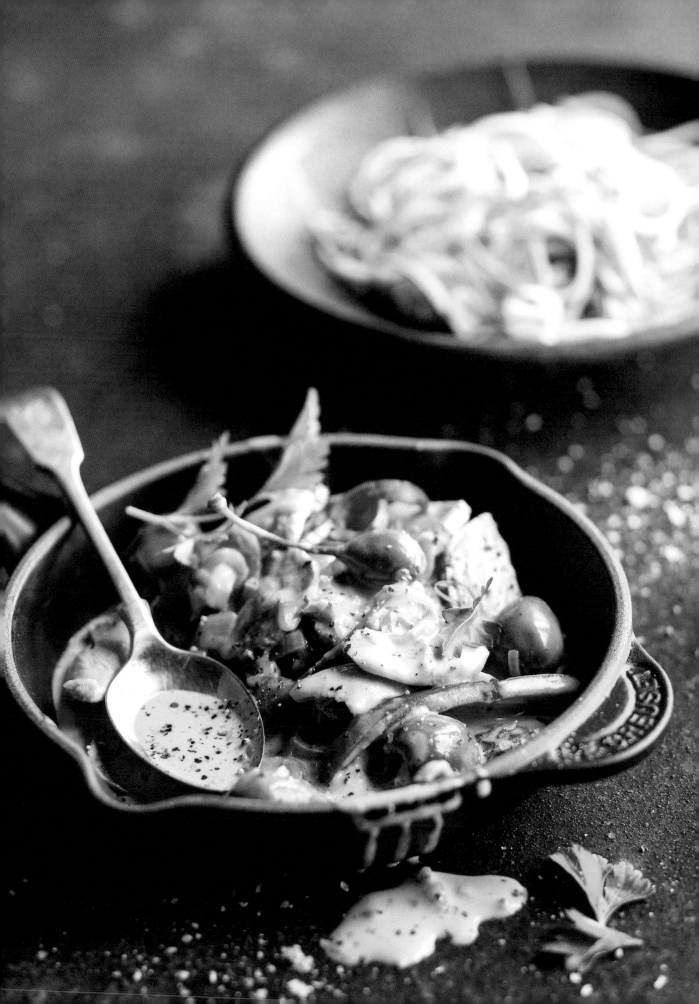

PONZU DUCK SALAD WITH CUCUMBER NOODLES

SERVES 2

Here we talk about 'noodles' for the first time. Giving up noodles leaves a lot to be desired in the way of texture in some of our favourite Asian dishes. But with a mandolin or Chinese slicer you can make 'spaghetti' out of almost any vegetable.

FOR THE DUCK

2 duck breasts

4 tbsp tamari soy sauce
(naturally fermented)

Salt and white pepper

FOR THE DRESSING

2 tbsp mirin

3 tbsp rice vinegar

1 tbsp tamari soy sauce

1 lime, juiced

¼ tsp toasted sesame oil

5 cm ginger, thinly sliced

FOR THE SALAD

½ daikon radish (or 5 little pink radishes), finely sliced

2 spring onions, finely sliced

6 mangetouts, finely sliced

3 cm ginger, finely sliced

Finely sliced chilli, to taste

½ cucumber, shredded or cut into noodles with a Chinese slicer or peeler

½ handful fresh coriander, chopped

★ Score the duck fat in a crisscross pattern with a very sharp knife, Stanley knife or scalpel.

★ Soak the duck breasts in soy sauce for about 15 minutes. Dry the duck completely using paper towels and season with salt and pepper.

★ In a pan, seal the duck breasts on a medium heat. Seal them skin side down first. Keep them on the skin until the fat has completely rendered out, then flip them and continue cooking until they are medium, about 8–10 minutes in total.

★ Rest the duck for about 3 minutes then slice as thinly as you can.

★ Combine all the dressing ingredients in a bowl. Add the duck and the dressing to the salad ingredients and toss gently. Serve immediately.

Note: Mandolins or Chinese slicers are available from Asian stores or online. We have used cucumbers here, but you could experiment with whatever you like. If you can't get a Chinese slicer, you can use one of those shredder/julienne peelers, available in all good cookshops.

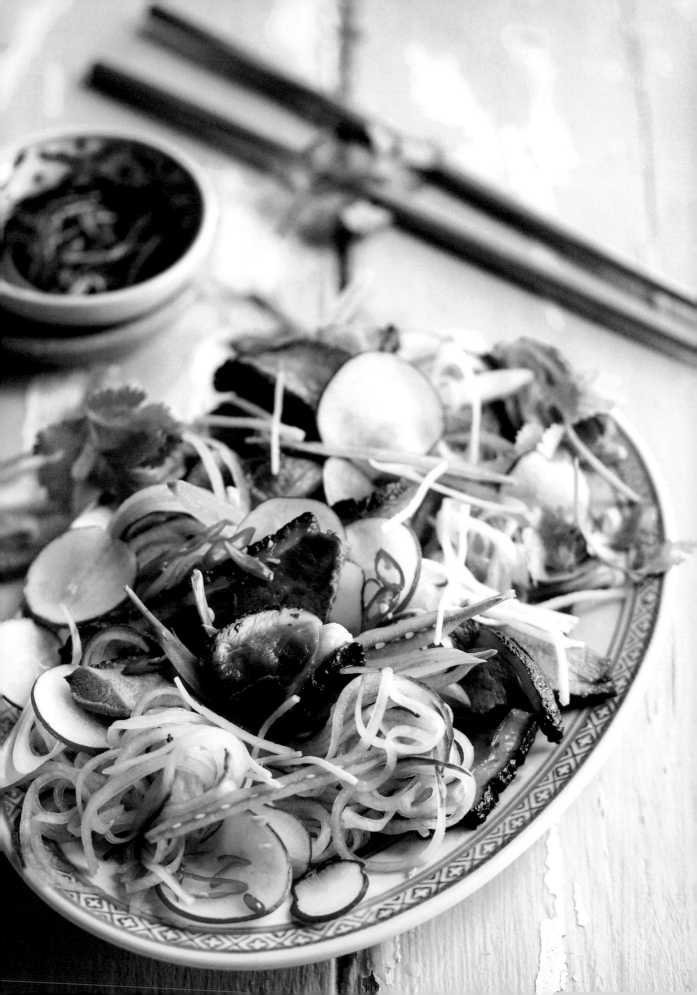

CHICKEN AND COCONUT BROTH

SERVES 4

1.2 l chicken stock

100 g mushrooms
(use wild mushrooms if
possible), sliced

2 sticks lemongrass, roughly
chopped

4 cm piece ginger, grated

1 red chilli, deseeded and
roughly chopped

400 ml coconut milk

2 tbsp fish sauce

2 tbsp lime juice, plus
wedges to serve

200 g cherry tomatoes,
cut in half

1 handful fresh coriander,
roughly chopped

★ Bring the stock to the boil in a medium-sized saucepan and
reduce it by half.

★ Add everything apart from the cherry tomatoes and
coriander to the stock and simmer for 10 to 15 minutes;
taste to check that all of the flavours have infused nicely.

★ Stir in the cherry tomatoes and simmer for about
five minutes.

★ Finally, sprinkle with coriander and serve immediately.

*Note: Thai seasoning comprises sweet, salty, spicy, bitter and
sour. Because of the restriction of sugar we have left it out of
the recipe but if you've had a good day, a quarter teaspoon
of palm sugar will electrify this broth. You could also use a
pinch of xylitol as a safer option. Try adding some shredded
chicken to this to make it more substantial.*

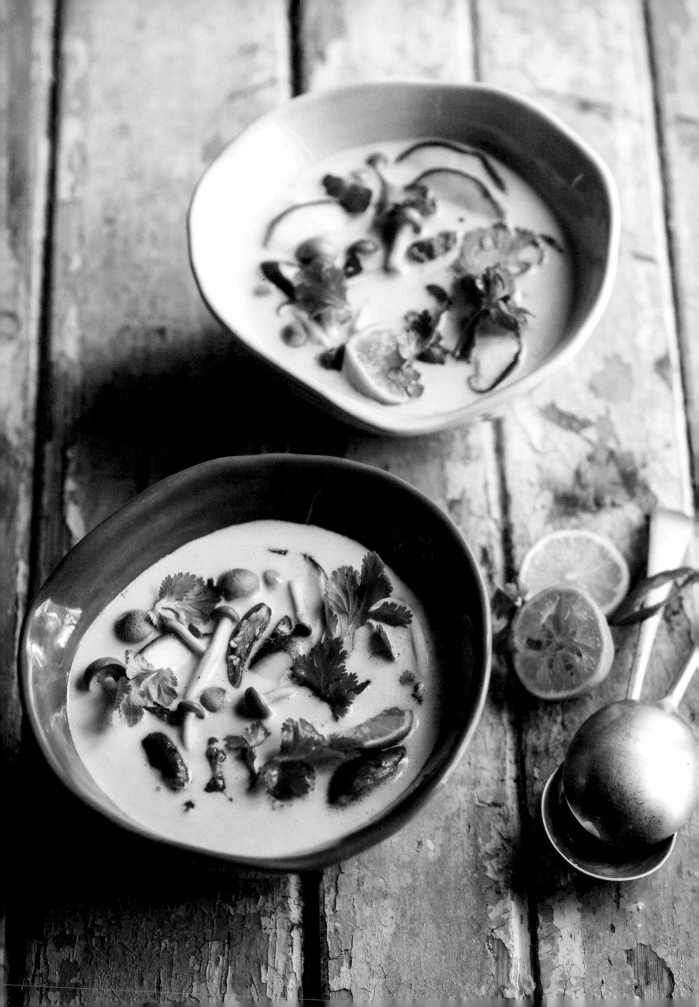

SPICY CHICKEN WINGS WITH BLUE CHEESE DIP

SERVES 6

'Buffalo Wings' are a classic American-style bar snack. Most of the time, the wings are drenched in a tangy marinade laced with sugar for those crispy sticky burnt bits. Here is a sugar-free version that we hope will guarantee the same satisfaction.

FOR THE BLUE CHEESE DIPPING SAUCE

50 g blue cheese (Stilton, Gorgonzola, Roquefort, etc.)

50 g cream cheese

200 ml buttermilk

1 handful parsley, chopped

1 small bunch chives, roughly chopped

Salt and pepper

FOR THE CHICKEN WINGS

3 cups Parmesan cheese, grated

3 tsp dried oregano

3 tsp paprika

3 tsp dried parsley

1 tsp dried chilli flakes

1 tsp salt

1 tsp ground black pepper

24 chicken wings, pointy bits removed and wings cut in half on the joint

250 g butter, melted

★ Preheat the oven to 180°C (Gas 4).

★ Make the blue cheese dipping sauce by blitzing all the ingredients together in a blender. Set aside.

★ In a bowl, mix the Parmesan, oregano, paprika, parsley, chilli flakes and salt and pepper. Dip each chicken wing in melted butter and then into this seasoning mixture and lay on a foil-lined tray ready for the oven.

★ Roast the wings until dark and crispy (roughly 40 minutes) and serve hot with the dipping sauce.

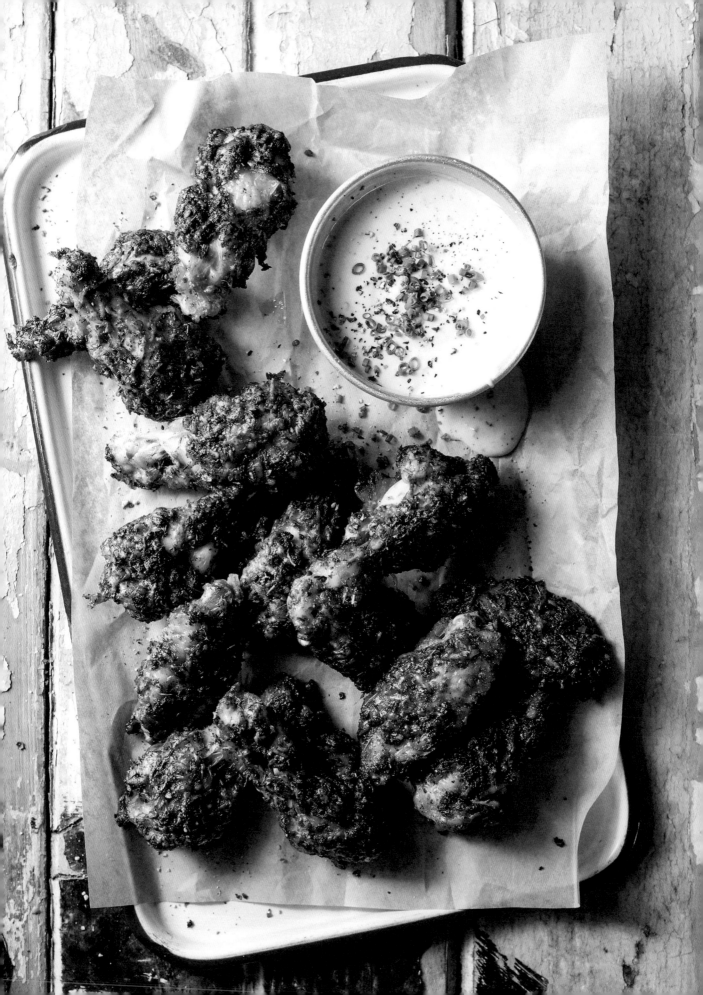

FISH AND SEAFOOD

I am absolutely obsessed with seafood. One of the best things about seafood is that it's pretty hard to get fish from the sea that isn't organic. The most important thing when buying seafood is making sure it is from a sustainable source and that the fish you are buying is what your fishmonger says it is. Most of these recipes are quick and dead simple. If complicated flavours confuse you, you're always safe with fish because 90 per cent of the time, all you need is salt and pepper and you're winning. The other bits and bobs are just for the hell of it!

Game fish ceviche

Trout carpaccio with celery and cucumber pickle and goats' cheese

Baked salmon with lemon, bacon and tomato

Warm haddock and cauliflower salad with tahini dressing

Herring, cucumber and fennel salad with a mustard and cream cheese dressing

Grilled salmon with caper noisette and wilted spinach

Tom yum prawn broth

Seared tuna with warm Italian umami salad

Thai steamed fish pocket

Grilled calamari with olives and cabanossi

Jamaican jerk baked fish with cucumber salsa

Margarita prawns

Steamed mussel pot

Fish soup with tomato and chorizo

Coconut-crumbed white fish with curry mayo

GAME FISH CEVICHE

SERVES 2

I think by now most people are used to ordering raw fish in sushi restaurants, but I know that many are still afraid to make it raw at home. I can assure you that your home kitchen is as clean and safe as any restaurant kitchen that cooked, or didn't cook, your fish. It is safe and brilliant. Game fish are fish such as salmon, tuna and swordfish. The only word of warning here is that some fish such as swordfish have unusually high mercury content so maybe don't go nuts on these if you're pregnant.

100 g cherry tomatoes, cut in half

2 lemons, juiced

1 lime, juiced

2 tbsp capers, roughly chopped

1 handful mint, picked, washed and chopped

1 handful dill, picked, washed and chopped

1 handful coriander, picked, washed and chopped

1 bunch spring onions, finely chopped

Plenty of salt and pepper

½ cup extra virgin olive oil

400 g freshest raw game fish (tuna, salmon, swordfish etc.), filleted, bones out, skin off

★ Combine all ingredients apart from the fish and leave to steep for 20 minutes.

★ Dice the fish into 1 cm cubes (you can ask your fishmonger to do this for you).

★ Cover the fish in ceviche marinade and leave to stand for 20 to 25 minutes in the fridge. The longer you leave it, the more the fish will 'cook' in the lemon and lime juice.

Note: Adding avocado to this seriously takes it up a notch.

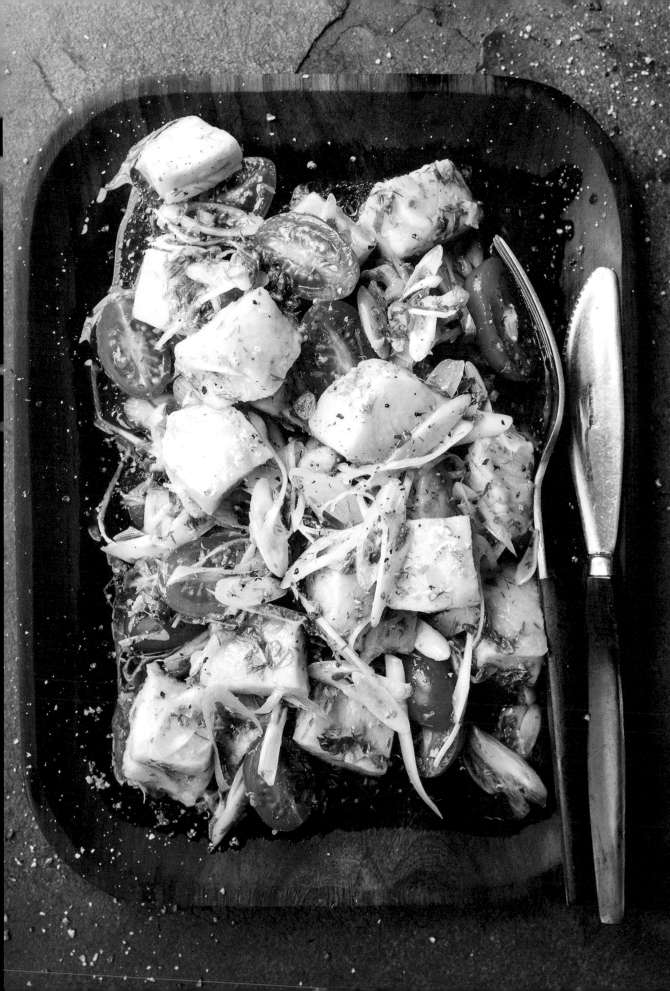

TROUT CARPACCIO WITH CELERY AND CUCUMBER PICKLE AND GOATS' CHEESE

SERVES 2

This is an excellent light lunch or starter dish. I love how the oily trout, creamy and sharp cheese and crunchy celery and cucumber pickle create such a great mix of texture in the mouth. The flavours here are seriously fresh and exhilarating.

¼ cucumber, shaved into long strips with a peeler

2 sticks celery, shaved into long strips with a peeler

1 lemon, juiced

3 tbsp apple cider vinegar

1 red chilli, deseeded and finely chopped

4 tbsp olive oil

200 g smoked trout ribbons, or thinly sliced very fresh raw trout

50 g chèvre (or any creamy goats' cheese)

★ Mix the cucumber, celery, lemon juice, vinegar, chilli and olive oil together in a bowl.

★ Lay the trout ribbons flat out on a plate.

★ Top the trout evenly with the celery and cucumber pickle. Break the goats' cheese into little pieces, dot it around the salad and serve.

Note: Leaving the pickle for about half an hour, if you have the time, really enhances the flavour.

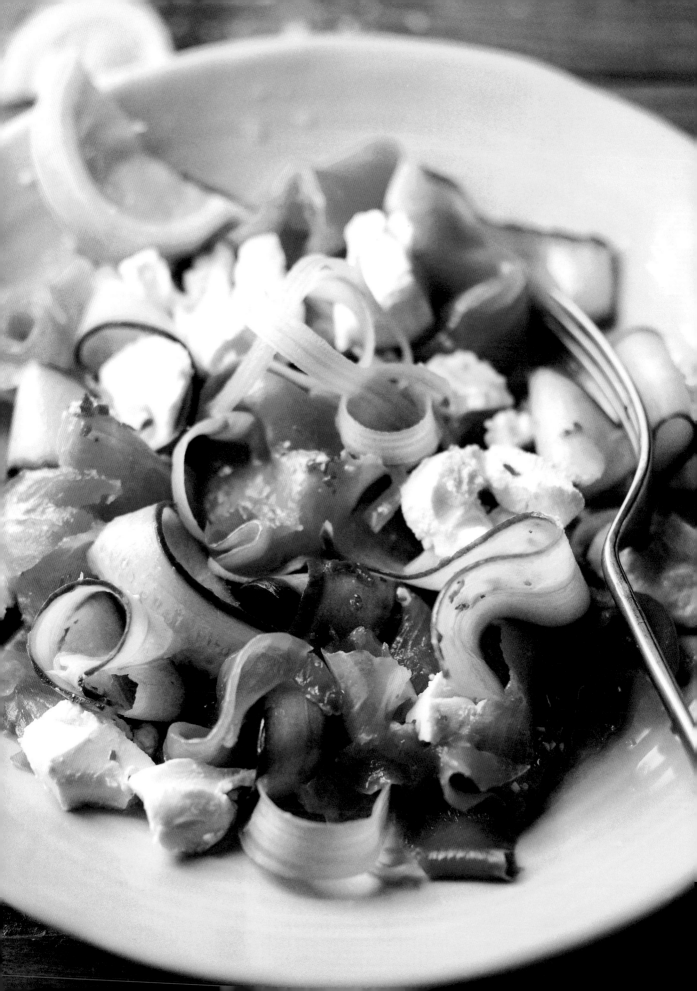

BAKED SALMON WITH LEMON, BACON AND TOMATO

SERVES 4

As we said earlier, we don't really like to mess with the flavour of a grilled piece of fish. If you make sure it's fresh, you've won half the battle already. One should be careful not to serve very strong flavoured accompaniments with the wrong fish as it could be completely over-shadowed. Without getting too technical, we will advise when you should use a game fish (much stronger in flavour, like salmon, trout or char) or a white fish (this is like hake or cod).

220 g good-quality bacon or pancetta, sliced into lardons

100 g butter

200 g cherry tomatoes, cut in half

1 large lemon, juiced and zested

1 cup white wine

1 big handful of basil, torn

1 kg side salmon, skin on, bones out

★ Preheat the oven to 180°C (Gas 4).

★ In a large pan, sauté the bacon in the butter until it begins to crisp.

★ Add the cherry tomatoes and lemon zest and crank the heat up onto high so they colour a bit.

★ Now, add the wine and lemon juice and let it reduce down by about half.

★ Add in a big handful of torn basil and stir while removing from the heat.

★ Place the fish in a well-greased oven dish and spoon the mixture from the pan evenly over it.

★ Bang the tray in the oven for about 20 minutes and then check the fish. You can tell if it is cooked by using a fork in the thickest part of the fillet to pull the meat to one side. If it flakes away nicely and is still moist, you're on the money!

Note: When cooking fish there are two schools of thought: cook it fast and hot and get lots of colour, but risk overcooking it, or cook it slowly on a low temperature and guarantee a perfect melt-in-the-mouth sensation. Some fancy restaurants cook fish at 70°C (158°F) and it literally does melt.

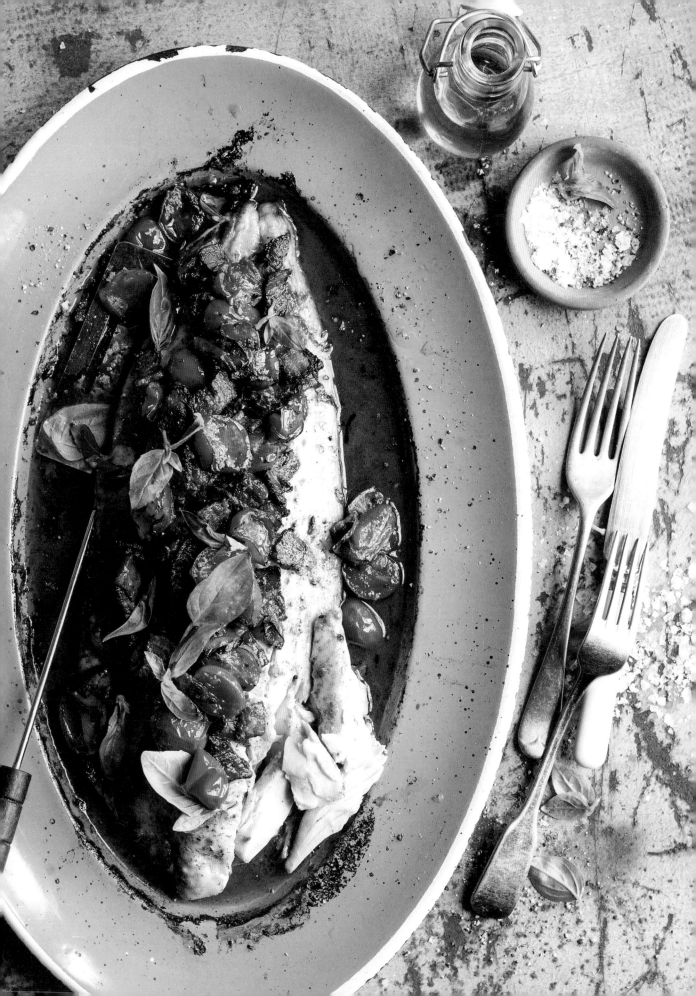

WARM HADDOCK AND CAULIFLOWER SALAD WITH TAHINI DRESSING

SERVES 2

Smoked haddock is another item I recommend having to hand. There are haddock dishes that work for every meal time – just make sure you buy undyed smoked haddock.

FOR THE DRESSING
4 tbsp tahini
Juice of 2 lemons
1 garlic clove, minced
¼ cup extra virgin olive oil
approx 100 ml water

FOR THE SALAD
100 g butter
300 g cauliflower, cut into small pieces
300 g smoked haddock
60 g toasted pine nuts

★ Preheat the oven to 180°C (Gas 4).

★ Melt the butter in the microwave or in a small pan. Place the cauliflower in a small oven tray and drizzle with butter.

★ Roast the cauliflower until it is golden on the edges, around 30 minutes.

★ Add the haddock to the tray and return to the oven for about 10 minutes.

★ Remove from the oven, break the haddock up and give everything a good mix, either in a bowl or in the tray.

★ Portion the salad onto plates and scatter with pine nuts.

★ Combine all the dressing ingredients together in a small bowl and while mixing continuously, pour in the water until you reach a good pouring consistency and drizzle over the salad before serving.

Note: if you've been good with your carbs for the day, this is epic with some pomegranate seeds scattered over it.

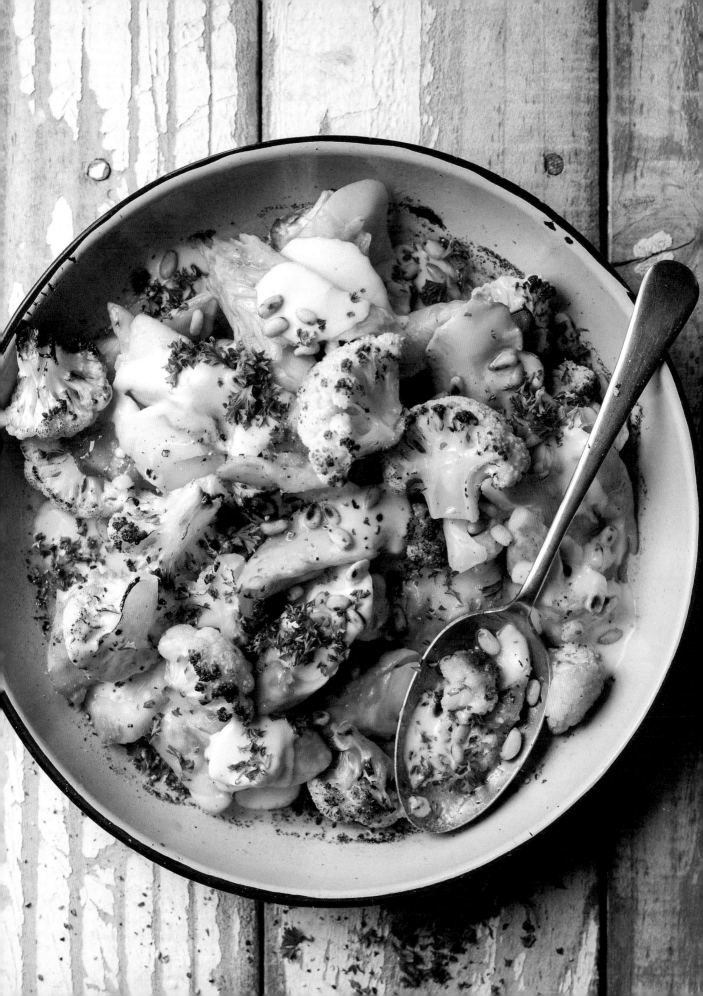

HERRING, CUCUMBER AND FENNEL SALAD WITH A MUSTARD AND CREAM CHEESE DRESSING

SERVES 2

I'm a big fan of pickled herring because its flavours are quite simple, making it pretty diverse. Herring comes in about a thousand formats so, honestly, you can use it however you like in this recipe.

FOR THE DRESSING

1½ tbsp wholegrain mustard

¼ cup thick cream cheese

Juice of 1 lemon

¾ cup milk

3 tbsp water

3 tbsp olive oil

1 handful chives, finely chopped

FOR THE SALAD

60 g wild rocket

½ large bulb fennel, finely shaved or sliced (reserve the fennel tops if you can)

¼ cucumber, shaved into strips with a peeler

1 tomato, cut into wedges (you can remove the seeds if you like)

200 g pickled herring

★ Combine all the dressing ingredients in a jug or bowl and blitz with a stick blender.

★ Lay the rocket out on a platter and scatter the fennel, cucumber, tomato and herring evenly over it.

★ Drizzle with the mustard dressing and serve immediately.

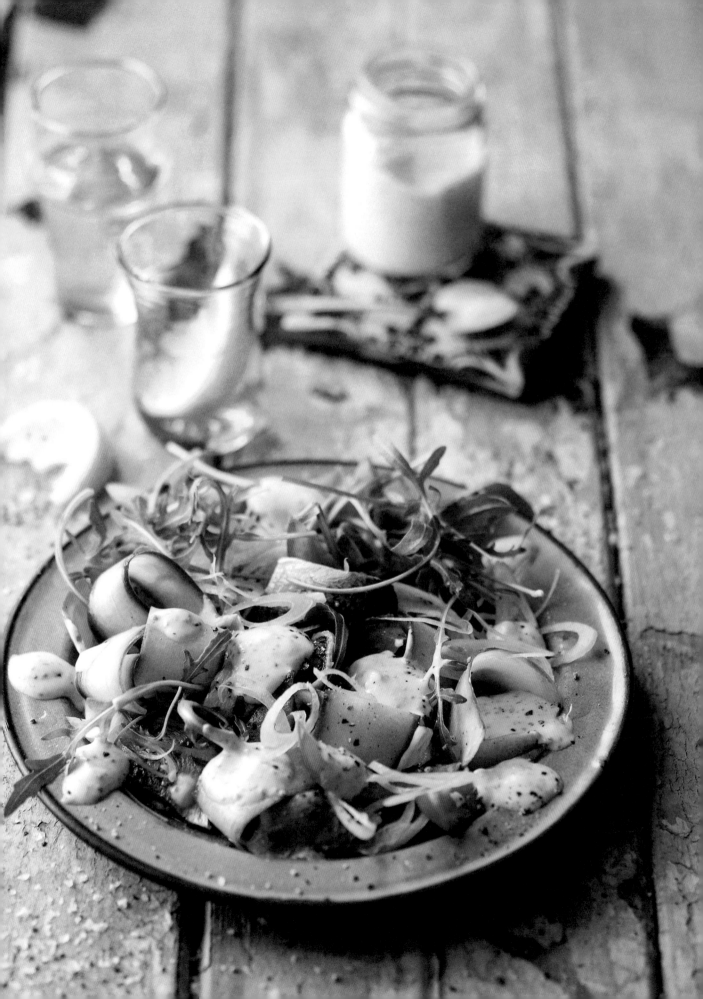

GRILLED SALMON WITH CAPER NOISETTE AND WILTED SPINACH

SERVES 2

'Noisette' is a French term used to describe a burnt-butter sauce, a classic accompaniment for fish that can be infused with a number of ingredients. The butter 'burns' when the clear and fatty component heats to a point hot enough to roast/toast/ burn the milk solids component. Clarified butter has a much higher burning point than normal butter.

FOR THE SALMON

2 portions salmon
(180 g each), skin on,
bones removed (or any other
oily fish)

Salt and pepper

100 g butter

3 tbsp capers
(rinsed and drained)

Zest and juice of 1 lemon

FOR THE WILTED SPINACH

50 g butter

200 g baby spinach, rinsed
well

Salt and pepper

★ Preheat the oven to 200°C (Gas 6).

★ Pat the salmon dry with paper towels and season liberally with salt and pepper.

★ Get a medium-sized heavy-based frying pan nice and hot and add in the butter.

★ Once the butter has melted and started to hiss and spit, add in the salmon, skin side down, in the pan.

★ Fry the salmon on its skin for about three minutes then gently lift the pieces and turn them (if your pan is the right heat, the skin will not stick). Fry for another three minutes on the other side before removing from the heat. It should be nice and pink (medium rare) on the inside. If you're not into raw fish, feel free to repeat another three minutes on each side until you reach the desired 'cookedness' or pop it in the oven for five minutes.

★ Once the salmon is out of the pan, add the capers and stir them around in the butter. When they begin to brown on the edges, add the zest of the lemons and then the juice and remove from the heat.

★ Melt the butter for the wilted spinach in a clean pan (or use the dirty salmon pan for extra flavour). Before the butter gets too hot, add in the spinach and stir on a high heat until completely wilted. Season with salt and pepper.

★ Serve the salmon on top of the wilted spinach and drizzle with the caper noisette.

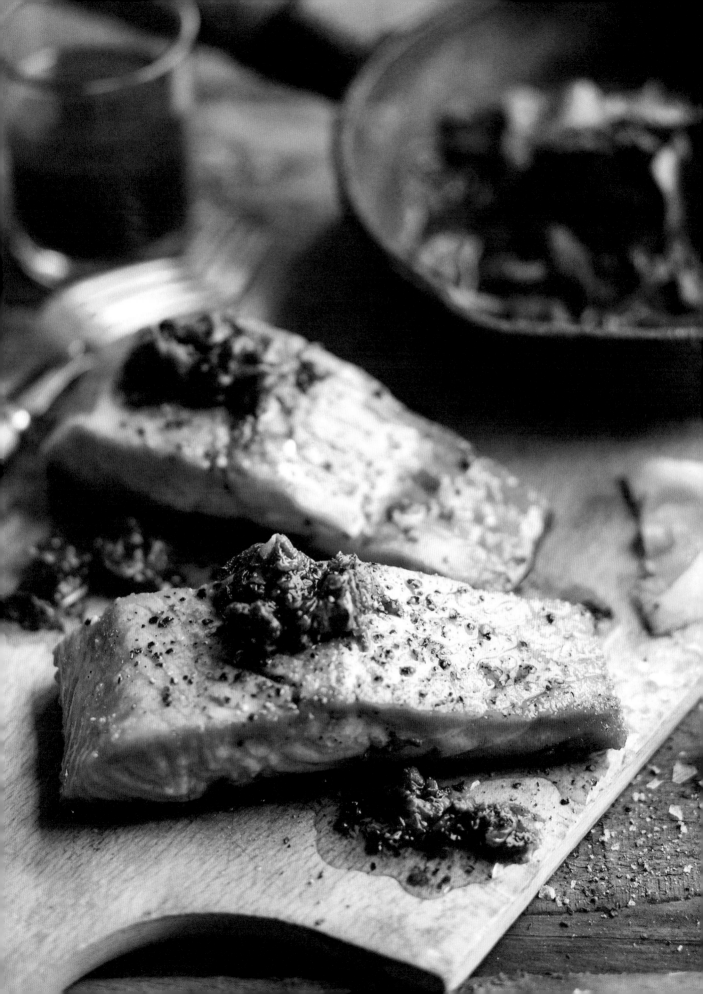

TOM YUM PRAWN BROTH

SERVES 2

In the West we use chicken stock but in Laos and Thailand they use stock from fish bones and prawn shells. Use whichever is easiest for you.

2 cups basic broth
(see page 64)

2 red chillies, deseeded and
cut in half down the middle

3 kaffir lime leaves

1 stick lemongrass, finely
chopped

1 large tomato, cut into
wedges

1 large flat mushroom, sliced

1 tbsp hot Thai chilli jam
or paste

Juice of 1 lime

3 tbsp fish sauce

250 g or 1 cup shelled and
deveined raw prawns

1 small bunch coriander

★ Combine all of the ingredients apart from the prawns and
the coriander in a pot and bring to the boil.

★ Simmer for 10 minutes, then add the prawns and coriander
and cook for just a couple of minutes until the prawns
are pink.

★ Balance the seasoning with lime juice and fish sauce and
serve as hot as possible.

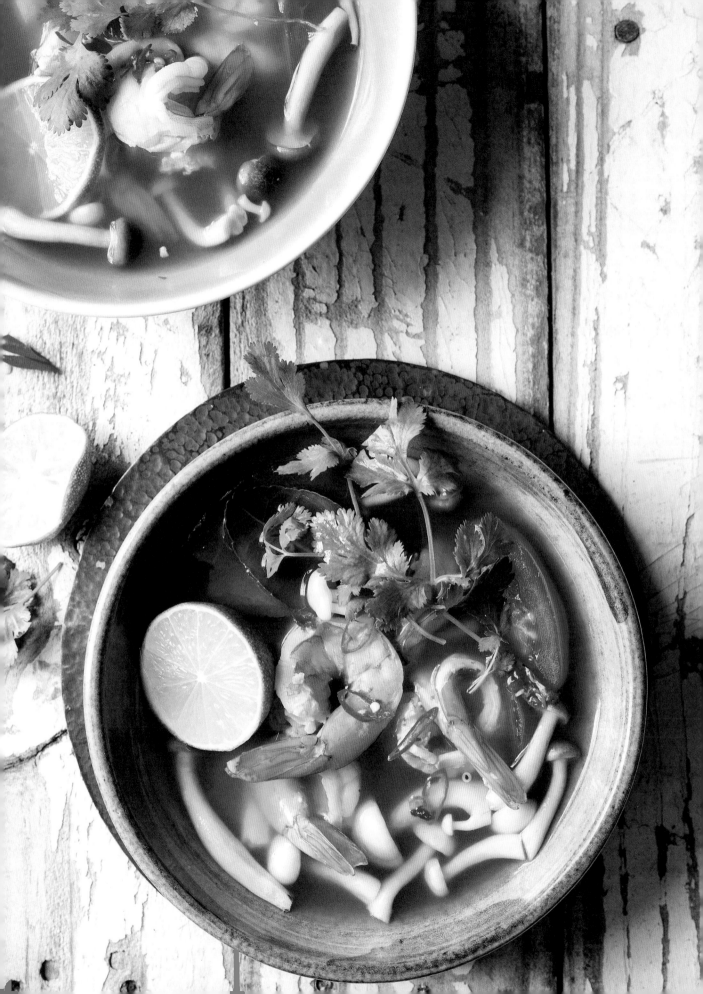

SEARED TUNA WITH WARM ITALIAN UMAMI SALAD

SERVES 2

Umami is supposedly the sixth flavour after sweet, sour, salty, spicy and bitter (these make up a lot of Asian flavours). It is the 'moreishness' you get out of food that contains MSG, soy sauce and a few other things. Until recently, I didn't know that parmesan is classed as the Mediterranean 'umami'. When you think about it, it makes sense! What doesn't taste good with Parmesan on it? Here's an Italian alternative to the standard Asian umami that we are used to!

3 tbsp good-quality anchovies, minced

Zest and juice of 2 lemons

1 cup cherry tomatoes, cut in half

1 yellow pepper, deseeded and cut into squares (the size of the cherry tomatoes)

1 tbsp capers, roughly chopped

1 red onion, sliced

¼ cup olive oil

2 garlic cloves, crushed

10 leaves basil, shredded

2 x 200 g tuna steaks

1 tbsp coconut oil for searing

80 g shaved Parmesan

★ Mix the ground anchovies and lemon zest into a paste to make the marinade.

★ Combine the lemon juice, tomatoes, pepper, capers, red onion, olive oil, garlic and basil together in a bowl.

★ Get a pan really hot and sear the tuna in the coconut oil for about 45 seconds on each side. If you like it well done, by all means cook it for longer.

★ Once the tuna is seared, remove it from the pan and smear it with the marinade.

★ Immediately add the mixture from the marinade bowl to the frying pan. Let it simmer, spit and boil for about 2 minutes. All of those flavours will come out beautifully!

★ Now, slice the tuna into bite-sized chunks.

★ Combine the tuna with the salad, top with Parmesan and serve immediately.

Note: If anchovies aren't your game, feel free to leave them out. They add to the umami but I know for a lot of people, they're a bit much.

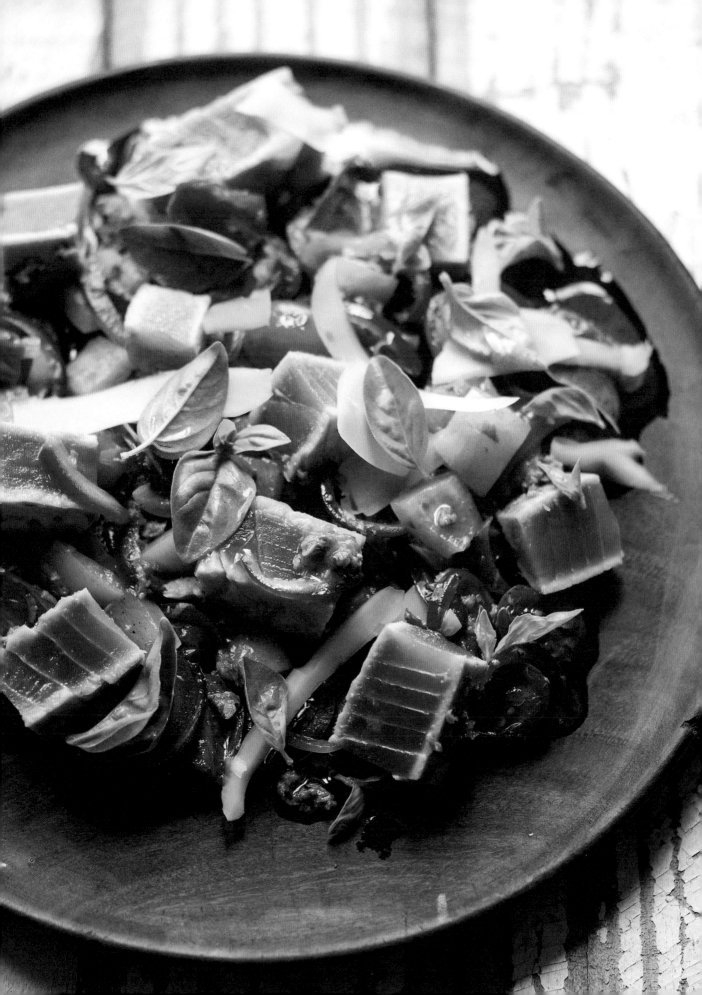

THAI STEAMED FISH POCKET

SERVES 2

A fish pocket is quite similar to poaching in that you are also able to penetrate the fish with flavour. You're also not bound to the indoor kitchen with pockets as they cook just as well directly on hot BBQ coals as they do in the oven.

200 ml coconut cream

2 limes

2 tbsp fish sauce

1 tbsp Thai chilli and garlic sauce

1 tsp red curry paste

2 spring onions, finely chopped

1 handful fresh coriander, roughly chopped

2 small heads bok choi, cut in half lengthways

2 x 200 g portions of white fish (hake, cod, pollock etc.)

★ In a bowl, combine everything apart from the bok choi and the fish.

★ Lay out two large sheets of heavy-duty aluminium foil. Top each large sheet with a similar-sized sheet of greaseproof paper or baking parchment.

★ In the centre of each sheet, place two pieces of bok choi.

★ Place a fish portion on top of each one and raise the edges of the foil to create a bowl.

★ Pour half of the sauce into each 'bowl' and scrunch the sides together to close the pocket.

★ Place this in a preheated oven at 200°C (Gas 6) for 12 minutes, or directly on the BBQ coals for 8 minutes.

★ Serve and pour the sauce from the pocket over the fish.

Note: you can use the same sauce pocket recipe with prawns or mussels.

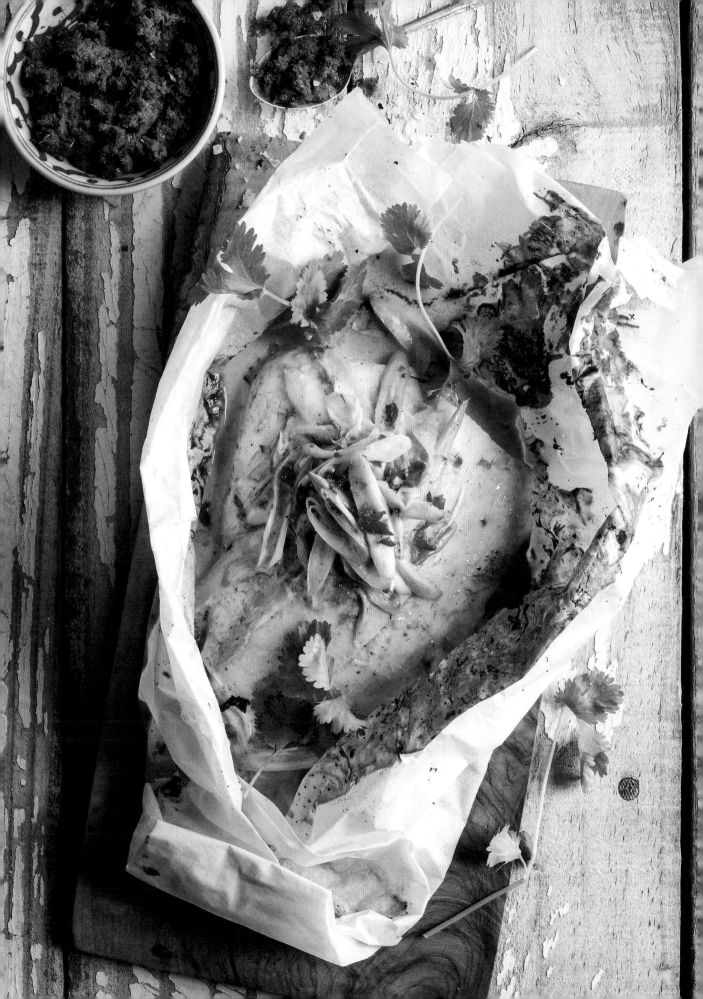

GRILLED CALAMARI WITH OLIVES AND CABANOSSI

SERVES 2

If you can get clean baby calamari, this dish can literally be finished in 10 minutes! Your fishmonger can do this for you. Cabanossi is a salami sausage popular in South Africa, but if you can't get it then any good-quality salami would work.

100g slices cabanossi

½ cup marinated green or black olives

1 red pepper, deseeded and finely diced

280 g cleaned baby calamari tubes and tentacles

2 garlic cloves, minced

1 lemon, juiced

1 bunch flat-leaf parsley, chopped

Salt and pepper

★ In a large heavy-based pan, sauté the cabanossi in its own fat with the olives on a medium heat until crispy.

★ Remove the olives and cabanossi but leave the fat in the pan.

★ Pump the heat up to full and wait for it to be smoking hot.

★ Add the pepper and give it a stir, then quickly add the calamari and leave it for a minute or so to colour. DO NOT STIR.

★ After a minute, you can move it around a little and toss the calamari on to their other sides.

★ Once the calamari begins colouring, add the garlic, olives and cabanossi and toss again.

★ Finally, add the lemon juice and parsley and season with salt and pepper.

Note: You could also add a small knob of butter at the end, which would bring the flavours together brilliantly.

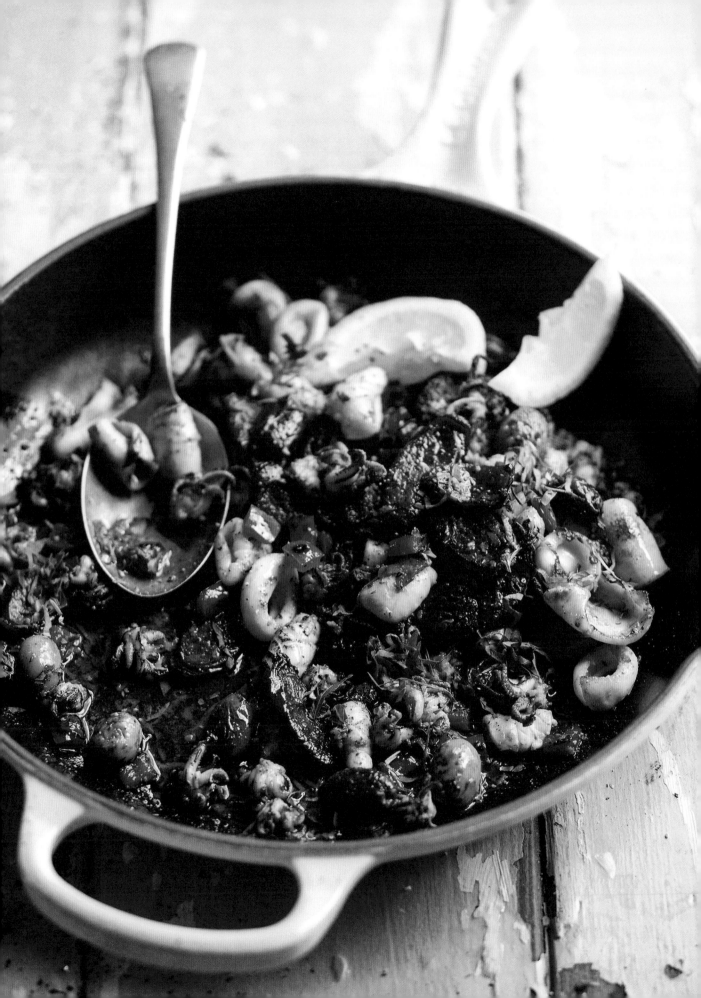

JAMAICAN JERK BAKED FISH WITH CUCUMBER SALSA

SERVES 4

We're not huge advocates for alcoholic consumption but there is some liquor that adds incredible flavour that we can't get anywhere else. Dark rum is one of those unique flavours. The good news is that when this marinade cooks, all of the alcohol will evaporate, so it's fine for everyone.

FOR THE JERK FISH

1 tbsp allspice berries

1 tbsp black peppercorns

½ tsp cinnamon

½ tsp cayenne pepper

2 tsp xylitol

2 bay leaves

1 large pinch ground cloves

2 tbsp thyme, picked and chopped

A few sprigs fresh coriander, chopped

1 red chilli, deseeded and finely chopped

1 garlic clove, finely chopped

1 knob ginger, grated

1 small bunch spring onions, finely chopped

Juice and zest of a lime

A splash of olive oil

2 tbsp dark rum (optional)

4 x 200 g portions fresh white fish (cod, hake, pollock, etc.)

FOR THE CUCUMBER SALSA

½ cucumber, finely diced

2 sticks celery, finely diced

1 red onion, finely chopped

3 radishes, thinly sliced

Juice of 1 lime

4 tablespoons olive oil

A handful chopped mint

Salt and pepper

★ Preheat the oven to 200ºC (Gas 6).

★ Combine all of the jerk ingredients (apart from the fish) in a food processor and blitz until smooth.

★ Massage the paste into the fish and leave to marinate for about 30 minutes.

★ Place the fish on a tray and bake for 10 minutes.

★ While the fish cooks, make the salsa by combining all of the ingredients in a bowl and mix well.

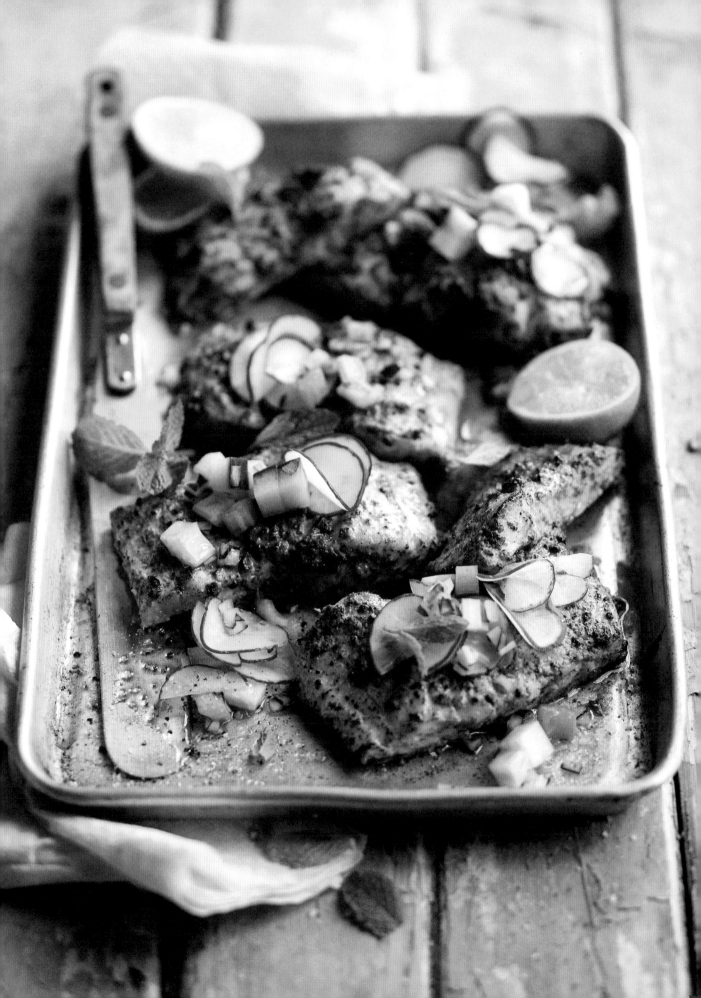

MARGARITA PRAWNS

SERVES 2

As we have mentioned before, alcohol is a touchy subject when it comes to drinking it. Cooking with it, however, opens the doors to a million more flavours. I highly recommend you use gold tequila for this dish as silver tequilas lack depth and complexity. Go for gold!

2 tsp dried mint

2 tsp dried dill

¼ tsp dried chilli flakes

Zest and juice of 1 big fat juicy lime

¼ tsp salt

12 large prawns, head on, shell on, butterflied

6 tbsp butter, divided in two

1 shot golden tequila

1 red chilli, deseeded and chopped

1 handful fresh coriander

Salt and pepper

★ Combine the mint, dill, dried chilli, lime zest and ¼ teaspoon salt in a small bowl to make the seasoning mixture.

★ Pat the prawns dry with paper towels and rub the seasoning mixture into the tail meat.

★ Get a large frying pan very hot and add in half the butter.

★ Once the butter is sizzling, add in the prawns, pump up the heat, and let them colour slightly on both sides.

★ After about four or five minutes, the prawns should be almost cooked. Now, pour in the tequila and flambé (either by lighting it with a lighter or briefly tilting the pan over the gas flames).

★ Once the alcohol has burnt off, add in the lime juice, the chilli, the remaining butter and the handful of coriander. Keep moving the pan so the butter emulsifies as it melts.

★ Finally, season with salt and pepper and serve.

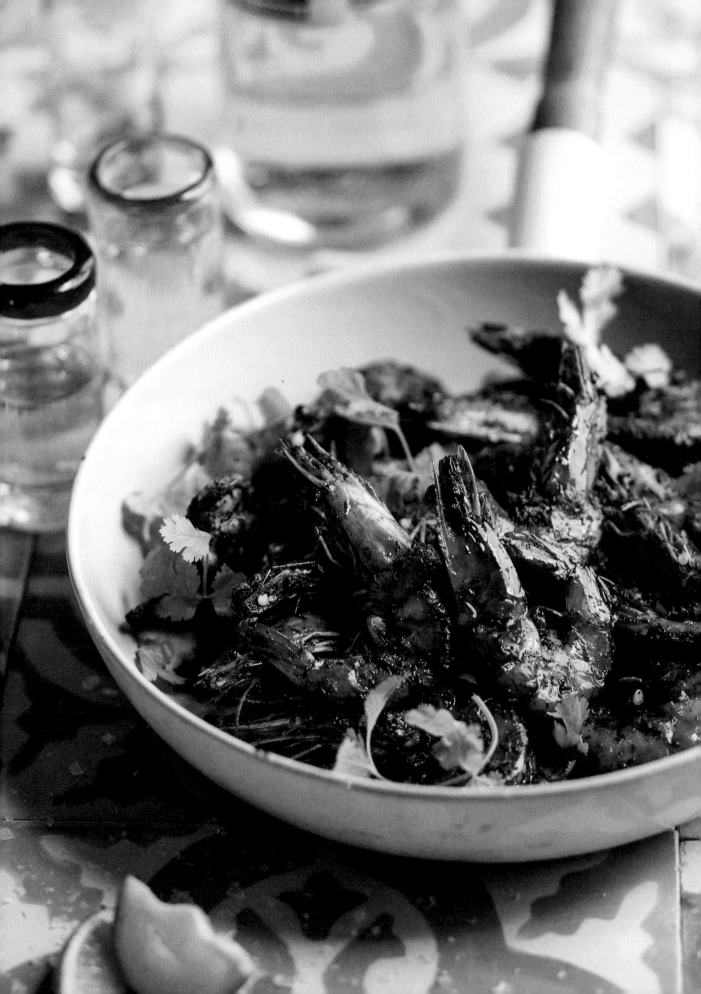

STEAMED MUSSEL POT

SERVES 2

This dish is a personal favourite of mine. Our family has a holiday house just outside Cape Town in South Africa. Every spring tide, we head down to a secret little cove just near the house and pick the mussels straight from the rocks. They are just so awesome when they're fresh like that.

2 tbsp butter

3 garlic cloves, sliced

1 knob ginger, grated

4 lime leaves

200 ml fish stock

2 green chillies, deseeded and sliced

2 lemongrass stalks, halved and bruised

Juice of 3 limes

2 tbsp fish sauce

75 g butter

1 kg mussels, cleaned and de-bearded

2 handfuls fresh coriander

2 spring onions, thinly sliced

★ In a shallow pot, melt 2 tbsp butter and gently fry the garlic and ginger until softened.

★ Add the lime leaves, fish stock, chillies and lemongrass and simmer for 5 minutes.

★ Add the lime juice, fish sauce and the mussels. Put the lid on and let the mussels simmer for 5 minutes until they start to open.

★ With a slotted spoon, spoon the mussels into a bowl, leaving the sauce in the pot.

★ Let the sauce cook down for 5 minutes then take the pot off the heat and whisk in 75 g butter to thicken the sauce slightly.

★ Stir in the chopped coriander and spring onion, spoon the sauce over the mussels and serve.

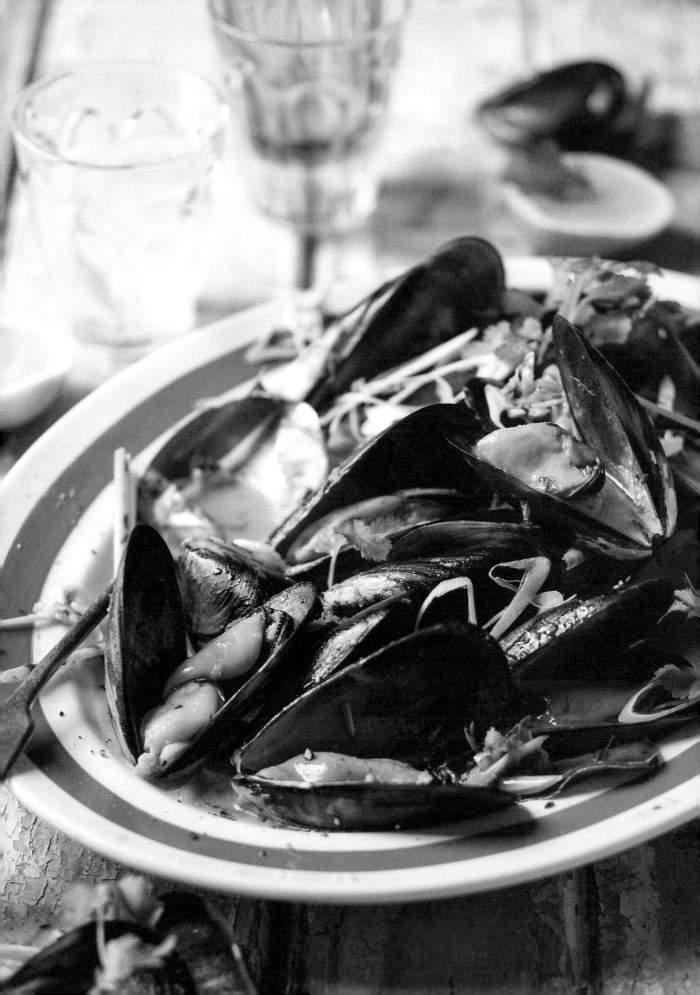

FISH SOUP WITH TOMATO AND CHORIZO

SERVES 2

1 knob butter

½ chorizo sausage, sliced

½ onion finely chopped

1 garlic clove, minced

2 stalks celery, finely diced

½ cup white wine

400 ml tomato passata

3 cups fish stock

300 g fresh cod, cut into cubes

1 handful flat-leaf parsley, picked and roughly chopped

1 handful fresh oregano, picked and roughly chopped

Salt and pepper

Juice of 1 lemon

★ In a large saucepan heat the butter and sauté the chorizo for three to four minutes.

★ Add the onion, garlic and celery and continue sautéing for three minutes.

★ Add the wine and reduce it by half.

★ Stir in the passata and stock, and simmer for 10 minutes.

★ Now, add the fish and simmer for another five minutes (or until the fish is cooked).

★ Finally, stir in the chopped parsley and oregano.

★ Season with salt, pepper and the lemon juice and serve immediately.

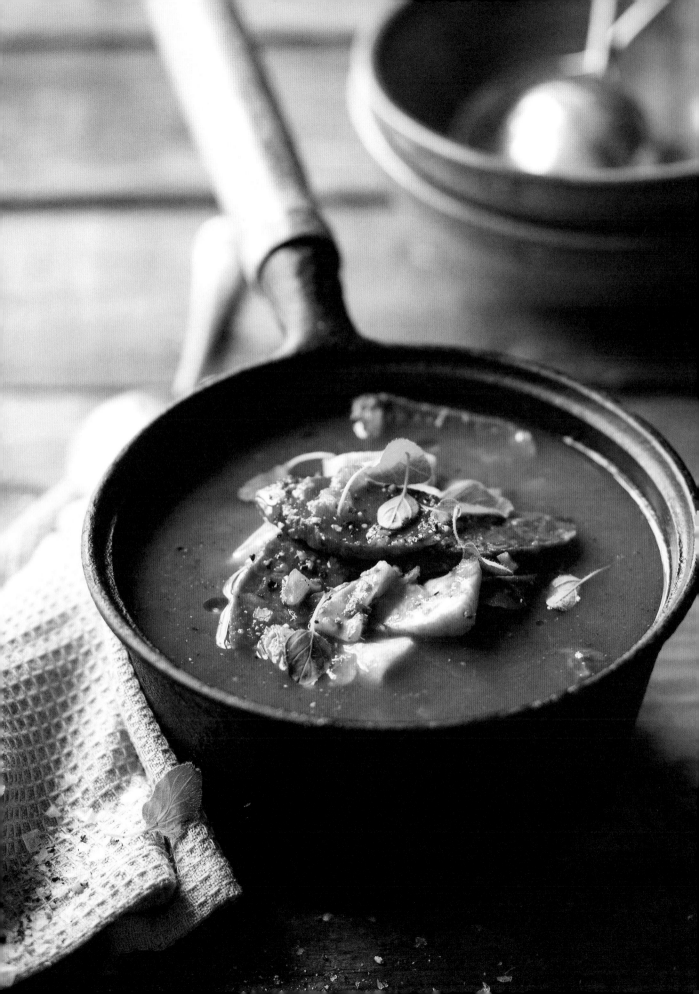

COCONUT-CRUMBED WHITE FISH WITH CURRY MAYO

MAKES 20 PIECES

In this recipe we teach you to crumb using desiccated coconut. If you have any recipes at home that call for breadcrumbs, you can swap them for desiccated coconut. They crisp up in exactly the same way as regular crumbs, only they offer a much nicer, nuttier flavour.

FOR THE CURRY MAYO

½ onion, sliced

2 tbsp butter

1½ tbsp curry powder

200 ml (one batch) Banting Mayonnaise (see page 66)

1 handful fresh coriander

Juice of 1 lime

Salt and pepper

FOR THE COCONUT-CRUMBED WHITE FISH

600 g clean white fish, skin off, bones out

2 eggs, beaten

1 cup desiccated coconut

80 g butter or coconut oil for frying

1 lemon, cut into wedges

Salt and pepper

★ Make the curry mayo. Sauté the onion in the butter until golden brown, then add the curry powder and fry until the aromas are released. Scrape the onion and curry mixture into a bowl with the mayonnaise and the remaining mayo ingredients. Blitz this with a stick blender and season to taste. To improve the flavour even more, add a tablespoon of crushed ginger and garlic to the onions while you fry the curry powder.

★ Cut the fish into 20–30 g strips.

★ Place the beaten egg in one dish and the coconut in another. Dip each strip of fish, one at a time, into the egg and then into the coconut. Place the crumbed pieces on a clean tray.

★ Melt the butter or coconut oil in a frying pan and pan-fry each piece until golden brown.

★ Drain on paper towels, season and serve hot with lemon wedges and the curry mayo.

Note: You can grill the fish in advance and warm them in the oven before serving for an easy way to make larger batches.

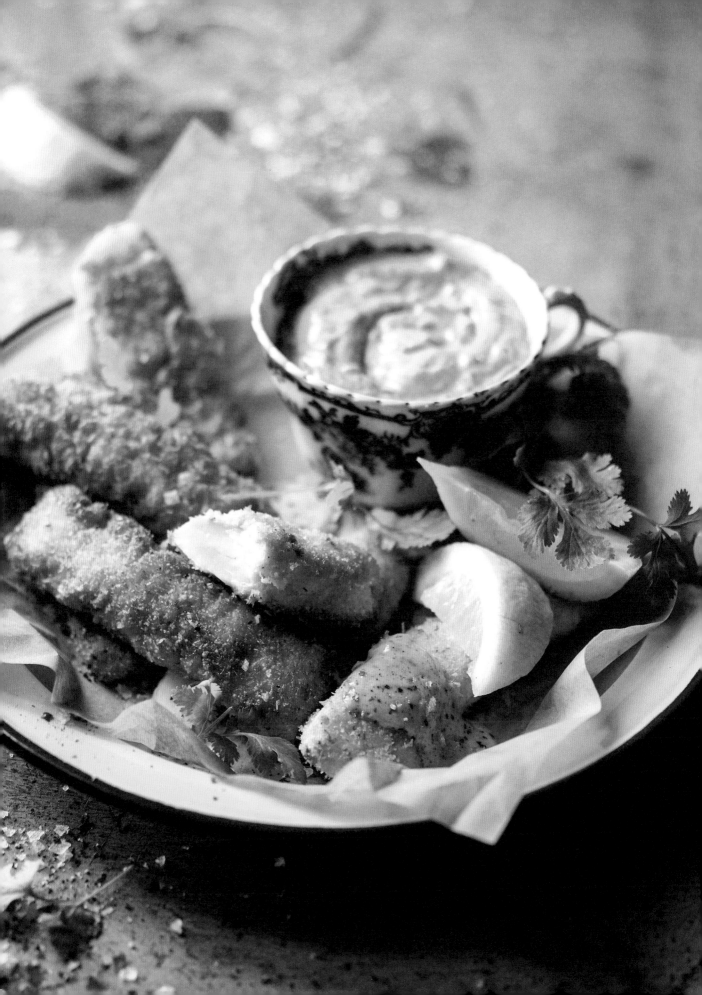

SIDES AND SALADS

Contrary to popular belief, vegetables still make up the biggest part of this way of eating. A lot of people think Banting is just fat and meat, but that's hogwash. The reason we shamelessly promote Banting is because the benefits of eating so many nutritious, low-carb veggies by far outweigh the benefits of eating rice and potatoes at every meal.

We've given you a decent mix of quick, medium and slightly more time-consuming recipes for vegetables. There are thousands of veggies out there so please don't use this as your strict guide. Swap ingredients in and out and match different sides with different meat and fish dishes. There are two golden rules we like to follow when planning a menu that you may find helpful.

Firstly, always make sure that, across the menu, you have a good mix of flavours that go well together. Following the flavours associated with a particular country always helps; for example, if you had tomatoes, cheese and basil in the fridge you could create the rest of your meal using other Italian ingredients and be completely safe in the knowledge that it would all work.

Secondly, keep in mind the textures that each dish or element will offer. To keep things exciting you always want to have a little crunch, something smooth or creamy and then something that offers a little more chew like a protein. So if you're serving mashed cauliflower, the last thing you would pair it with would be soft roasted aubergines. You would want to go with some crunchy steamed broccoli or al dente asparagus.

If you're trying a completely new vegetable and aren't sure what to do with it, always start by adding butter and bacon, and see how you go from there.

Asparagus, Parmesan, lemon and olive oil

Courgette and garlic gratin

Sage and blue cheese roasted squash

Buttered Brussels sprouts with bacon
and crème fraîche

Wilted onion and walnut spinach

Shiitake mushroom, bok choi and
mangetouts stir-fry

**Green beans with toasted almonds
and lemon butter**

Crunchy cabbage salad with creamy
red curry dressing

**Broccoli and avocado salad with
roasted almond dressing**

Avocado, sugar snap pea and mint salad with
poppy seed dressing

Marinated tomato and anchovy salad

Spiced pumpkin and goats' cheese,
sunflower seeds and citrus dressing

Charred halloumi and pepper salad

Charred aubergines with pine nuts and tahini

ASPARAGUS, PARMESAN, LEMON AND OLIVE OIL

SERVES 2

Asparagus has such good flavour that I don't dare to mess with it. This dish, and asparagus in general, goes brilliantly with beef, lamb and fish – and also does pretty well on its own.

300 g thick asparagus spears, woody stalks removed

Juice of 1 large lemon

40 g Parmigiano Reggiano

50 ml extra virgin olive oil

Salt and black pepper

★ In a small pot, bring some water to the boil.

★ Blanch the asparagus spears in the water for 2 minutes (or until they go bright green). Then refresh them in cold water, until cooled properly.

★ Lay the asparagus spears out on plates or a platter and sprinkle with lemon juice.

★ Shave or grate the Parmigiano Reggiano on top of them, being sure to coat well.

★ Splash with olive oil, season liberally with salt and pepper and serve.

Note: The success of this recipe lies in the freshness and quality of the Parmesan. Make sure you get Parmigiano Reggiano – no other cheese will cut it!

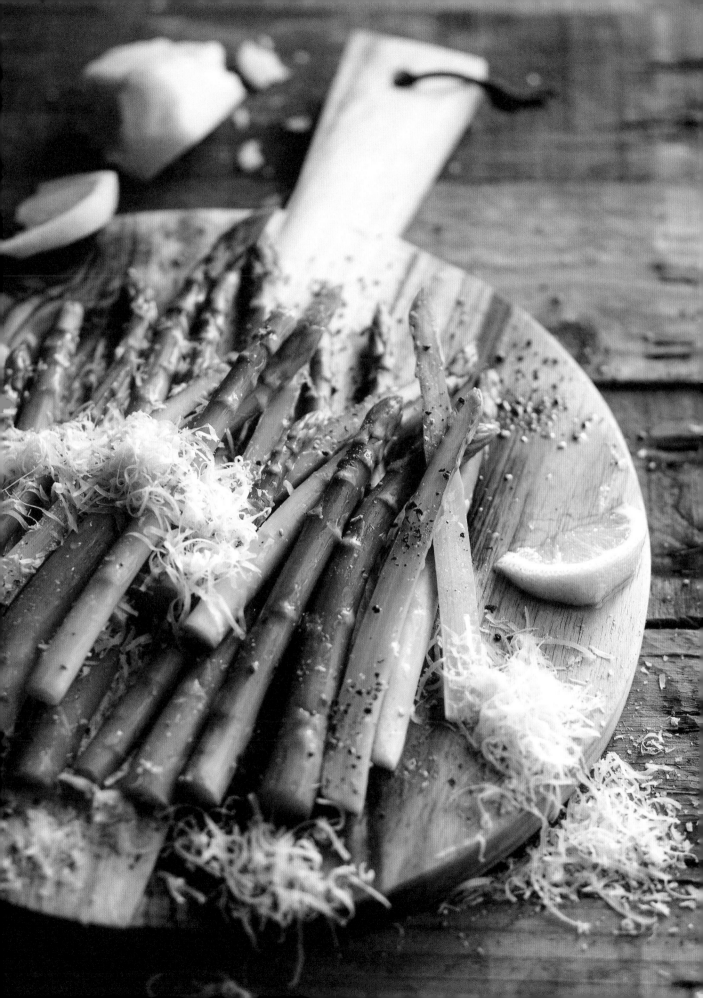

COURGETTE AND GARLIC GRATIN

SERVES 4

This is serious comfort food. It takes no time to prepare and stays in the oven for quite a while, so you can happily leave it to cook and forget about it until it's done.

800 g courgettes

1 onion, roughly sliced

1 handful thyme sprigs

1 whole head garlic, cloves peeled

100 g butter, broken into pieces

250 ml double cream

Salt and pepper

★ Preheat the oven to 200°C (Gas 6).

★ Cut the courgettes into large chunks.

★ Lay the onions, courgettes, thyme and garlic in an ovenproof lasagne dish (or casserole dish), mix well and then press down.

★ Dot pieces of butter evenly over the top of the dish, then cover everything with the double cream. Season with salt and pepper.

★ Place the tray in the oven, uncovered, and bake for approximately 45 minutes.

★ If you want to thicken the sauce in the bottom of the tray simply strain through a sieve and reduce it on the stove before pouring it back over.

Note: If you want some extra goodness, sprinkle a layer of grated cheese on top of the gratin before serving and pop it back under the grill for a cheesy crust.

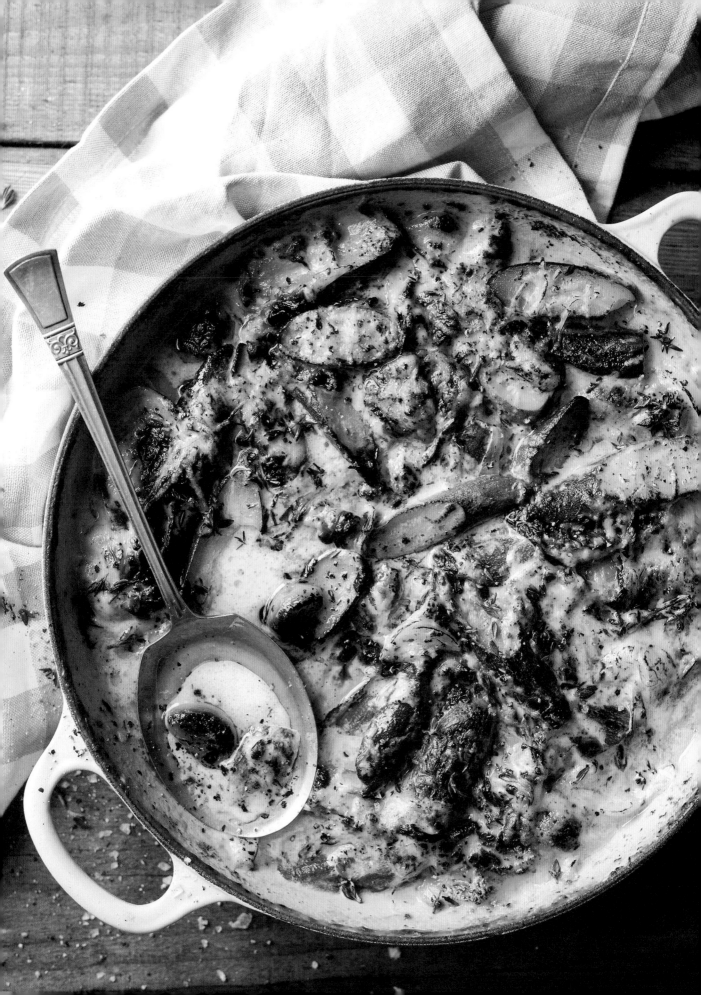

SAGE AND BLUE CHEESE ROASTED SQUASH

SERVES 4

While gem squash is not a particularly nutritious vegetable, adding a little blue cheese and some butter certainly gives it a little more excitement. This is gem squash at its most decadent.

4 small squash (round ones like acorn or gem) cut in half, seeds removed

150 g blue cheese

100 g butter

1 handful sage leaves

Salt and pepper

★ Steam or boil the squash until it is soft and tender (approx. 5–7 minutes).

★ Remove from the water and place in a tray.

★ Crumble an equal amount of blue cheese over each squash half.

★ Melt the butter in a pan and gently fry the sage until it goes golden.

★ Spoon the butter over each squash half and pop under the grill until the cheese is dark brown.

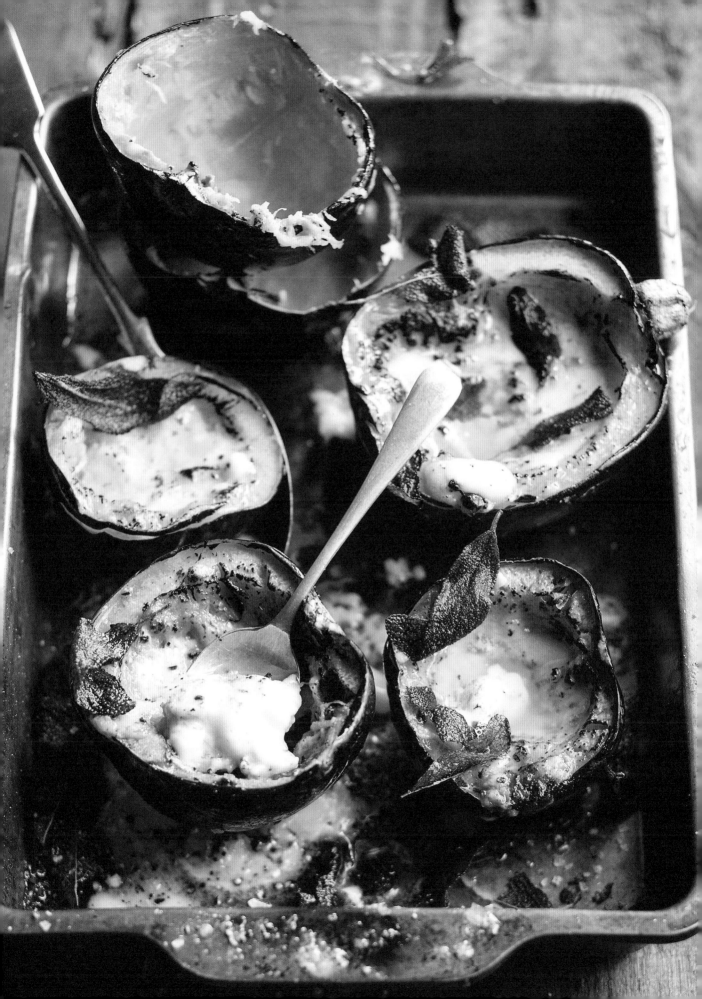

BUTTERED BRUSSELS SPROUTS WITH BACON AND CRÈME FRAÎCHE

SERVES 4

Personally, I'm not a huge fan of Brussels sprouts but I recently ate these at a restaurant in the Cape wine lands. True to the 'bacon + butter = delicious' formula, I absolutely loved them. I'd love to take credit here but I stole this idea from one of South Africa's greatest chefs, Bertus Basson of Overture in the Stellenbosch Winelands.

500 g Brussels sprouts

120 g streaky bacon, cut into lardons (little pieces)

40 g butter

100 g double-thick crème fraîche

Salt and pepper

★ In a small pot, steam the Brussels sprouts until they are soft (approx. 5 minutes).

★ In a heavy-based pan, sauté the bacon in the butter until it begins to go crispy.

★ Add the Brussels sprouts and toss in the bacon and butter to give them a good coating. Season to taste.

★ Keep cooking until the sprouts are warmed through and then serve immediately. Garnish with dollops of crème fraîche over the sprouts.

Note: You can convert this recipe to a bake by adding cream and leaving it in a tray in a preheated oven at 180°C (Gas 4) for about an hour.

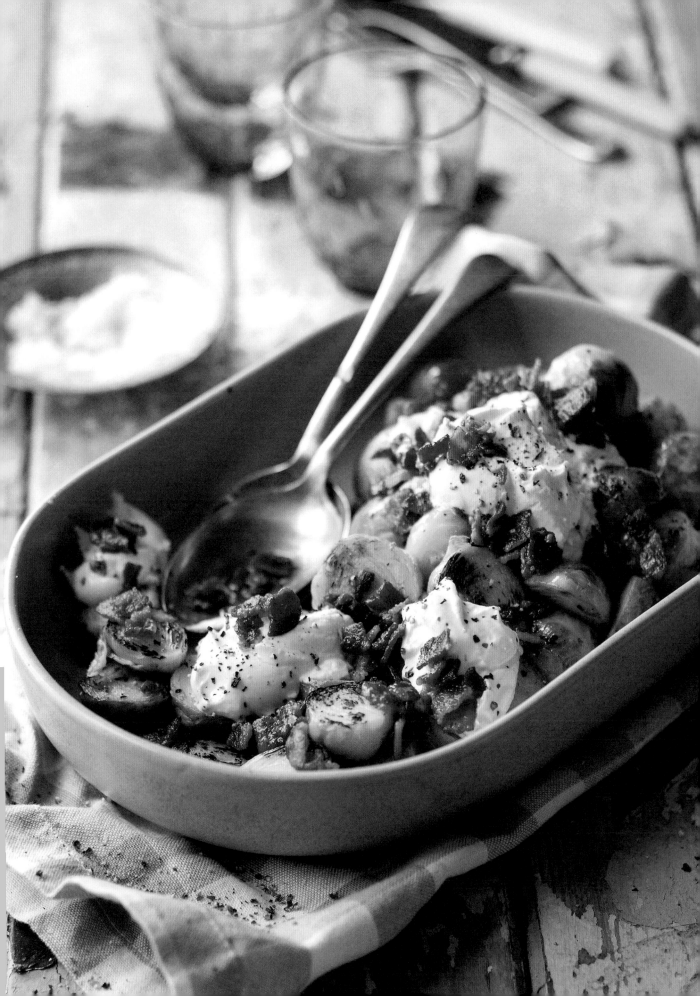

WILTED ONION AND WALNUT SPINACH

SERVES 2

This is actually a filling for a Middle-Eastern pastry called fatayer. *They are little pastry triangles that get served at all special occasions, in Lebanon especially. But it's just as delicious without the pastry – you could serve this with pretty much anything or eat it on its own.*

1 large onion, roughly
chopped

40 g butter

300 g baby spinach, washed
and roughly chopped

½ tsp sumac (optional)

Juice of 1 lemon

⅓ cup chopped walnuts,
toasted

Small bunch mint, finely
chopped

Salt and pepper

★ In a medium-sized pot, gently sauté the onions in butter until they go translucent.

★ Add the spinach and continue to stir until the spinach has cooked and any excess juice has evaporated.

★ Add the sumac (if using) and a squeeze of lemon, the walnuts and the mint; stir well.

★ Season to taste and serve now, or set aside for later.

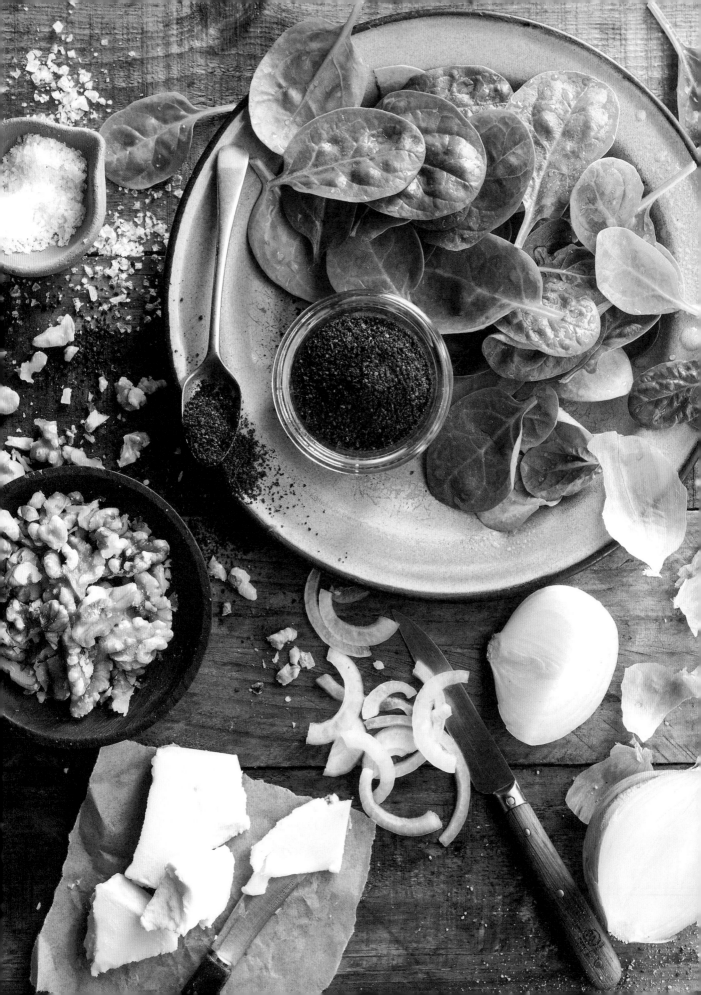

SHIITAKE MUSHROOM, BOK CHOI AND MANGETOUTS STIR-FRY

SERVES 4

1 tbsp coconut oil

2 garlic cloves, minced

5 cm ginger, peeled and grated

1 small chilli, deseeded and finely chopped

1 bunch spring onions, finely sliced

150 g fresh shiitake mushrooms, sliced

200 g mangetouts, cut in half lengthways

200 g baby bok choi, thickly sliced

1 tbsp fish sauce

2 tbsp mirin

Juice of 1 lime

1 large handful basil, roughly chopped

2 tbsp sesame seeds, toasted

★ Heat the coconut oil in a wok over a high heat.

★ As the oil begins smoking, add the garlic, ginger, chilli and the spring onions and stir.

★ Before the garlic starts colouring, add the mushrooms and sauté them for about two minutes, stirring constantly.

★ Once they are cooked, add the mangetouts and sauté until they go bright green.

★ Finally add the bok choi and cook until wilted.

★ Season with the fish sauce, mirin and lime juice. Mix through the basil leaves and the sesame seeds; serve.

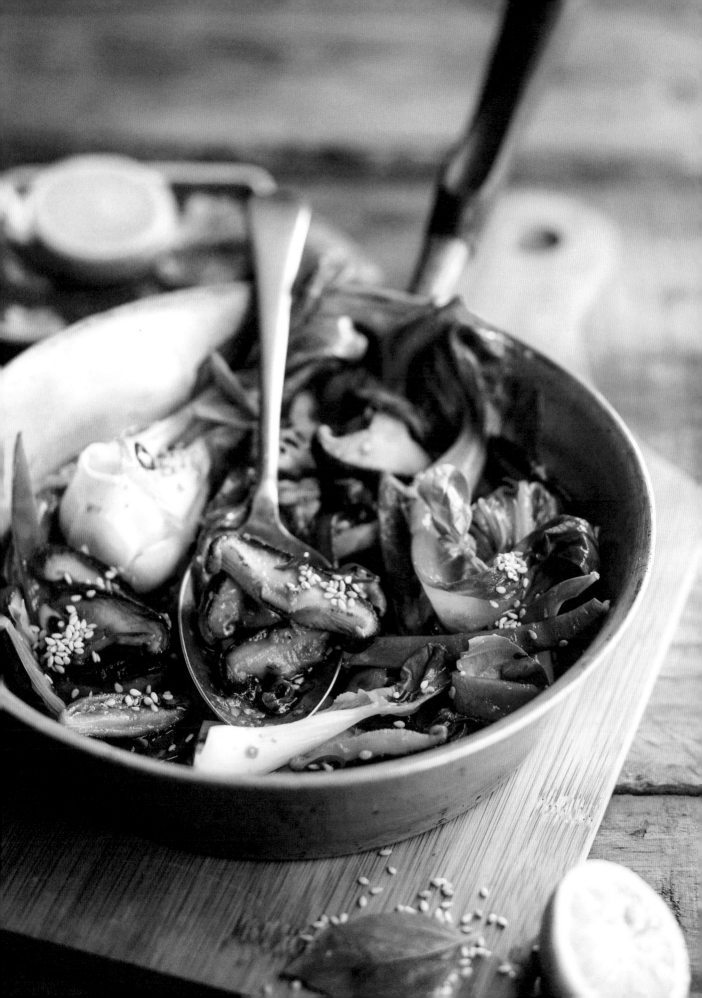

GREEN BEANS WITH TOASTED ALMONDS AND LEMON BUTTER

SERVES 4

Green beans and almonds is a classic French combination that is used as a side dish in a lot of restaurants. This dish pairs pretty well with anything simple like a grilled piece of meat or fish.

400 g green beans, topped and tailed

60 g butter

3 tbsp almond slivers, toasted in a dry pan

Juice of 1 lemon

Salt and pepper

★ Bring some water to the boil in a small pot and blanch the beans for 2 minutes. Refresh them in cold or iced water so they keep their colour and texture.

★ In a large pan or wok, melt the butter and warm it until just before it goes brown and add the beans (if it goes a little brown, it will add a nice nutty flavour).

★ Toss the beans until they are warmed through again, then add the almonds and the lemon juice.

★ Season with salt and pepper and serve.

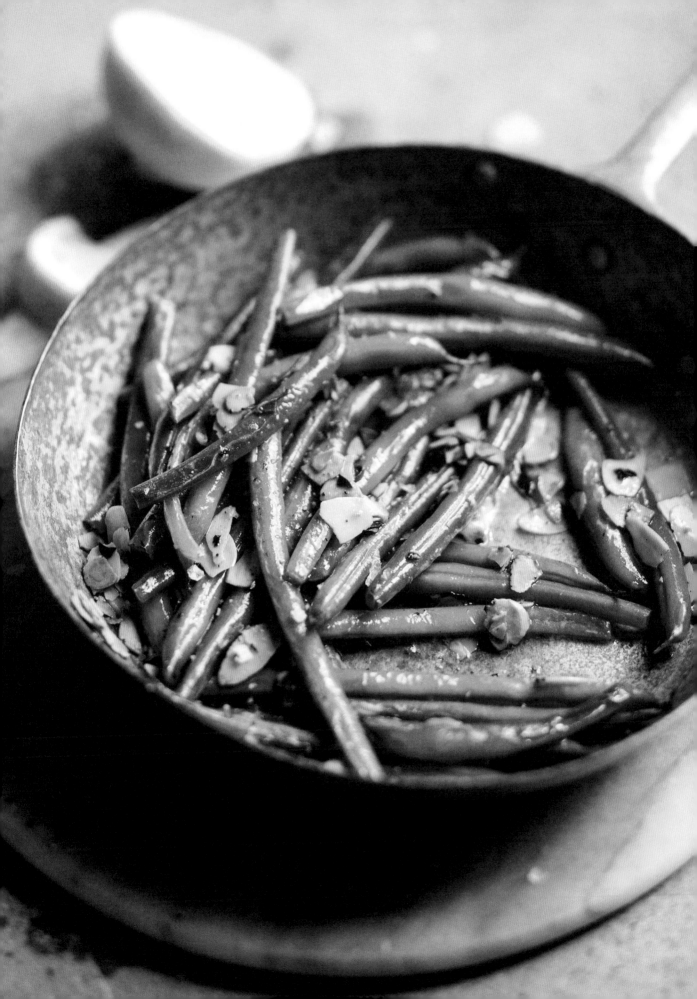

CRUNCHY CABBAGE SALAD WITH CREAMY RED CURRY DRESSING

SERVES 4

Cabbage is one of the most underrated salad leaves out there. It's dirt cheap and packed with tangy peppery flavour. This recipe strays from the standard coleslaw recipe as we want show you how cabbage holds its own against much more exciting flavours.

FOR THE DRESSING

1 tsp red Thai curry paste

1 tbsp lime juice

1 tbsp fish sauce

150 ml coconut cream

2 tbsp macadamia nut butter

1 handful fresh coriander, roughly chopped

FOR THE SALAD

½ white cabbage, shredded

1½ cups bean sprouts

1 bunch spring onions

1 cup toasted macadamia nuts (other nuts will be OK, just keep an eye on the carbs)

★ Make the dressing. Place all of the ingredients in a small saucepan and bring to the boil. Set aside and leave to cool.

★ Combine all of the salad ingredients in a mixing bowl and cover in dressing. Mix everything together and serve immediately.

Note: In Thailand, they don't generally use salt and pepper. Traditionally they season with lime juice (for acidity), fish sauce (which is salty) and palm sugar (for sweetness), so if you don't have lime juice or fish sauce you could always just add a squeeze of lemon and some salt to get the flavour right. Use xylitol for sweetness if you like.

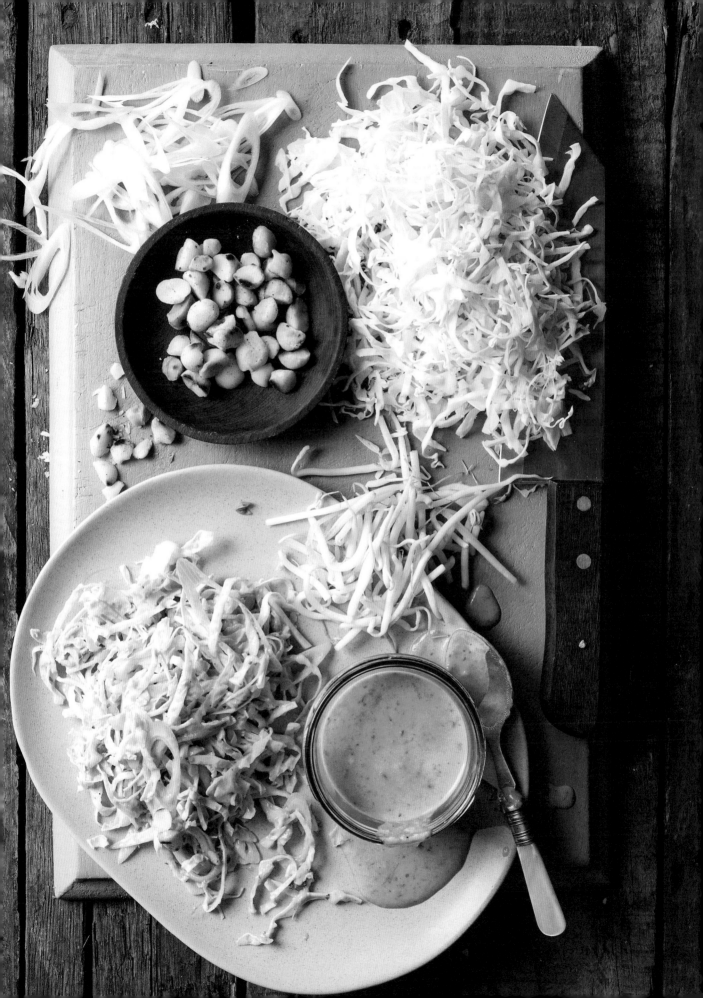

BROCCOLI AND AVOCADO SALAD WITH ROASTED ALMOND DRESSING

SERVES 4

This is another very simple, yet deliciously creamy, salad recipe.

FOR THE DRESSING

½ cup whole almonds

3 tbsp red wine vinegar

1 tbsp wholegrain mustard

4 tbsp crème fraîche

100 ml milk
Salt and pepper

FOR THE SALAD

400 g tenderstem broccoli
(you could use normal
broccoli, broken up into
florets)

2 ripe avocados, pitted and
cut into chunks

1 bunch spring onions,
finely sliced

1 small bag wild rocket

★ Make the dressing. Roast the almonds in the oven at 180°C (Gas 4) or toast under the grill until they are golden brown, then chop them up roughly. Add the remaining ingredients and half of the nuts to a tall narrow container and blend using a stick blender. Then stir in the remaining nuts and season to taste.

★ In a small pot of boiling salted water, blanch the broccoli until al dente (still crunchy) and refresh it in cold water.

★ Combine the broccoli, avocados, spring onions and wild rocket, mix gently and spread over a platter.

★ Pour the dressing over the salad and serve.

Note: Make sure the dressing has cooled before pouring it over the salad as it may discolour the avocado. We blend only half of the nuts because they help make the dressing creamy and the flavour infuses better that way. The second addition of crushed nuts is for some crunchy texture.

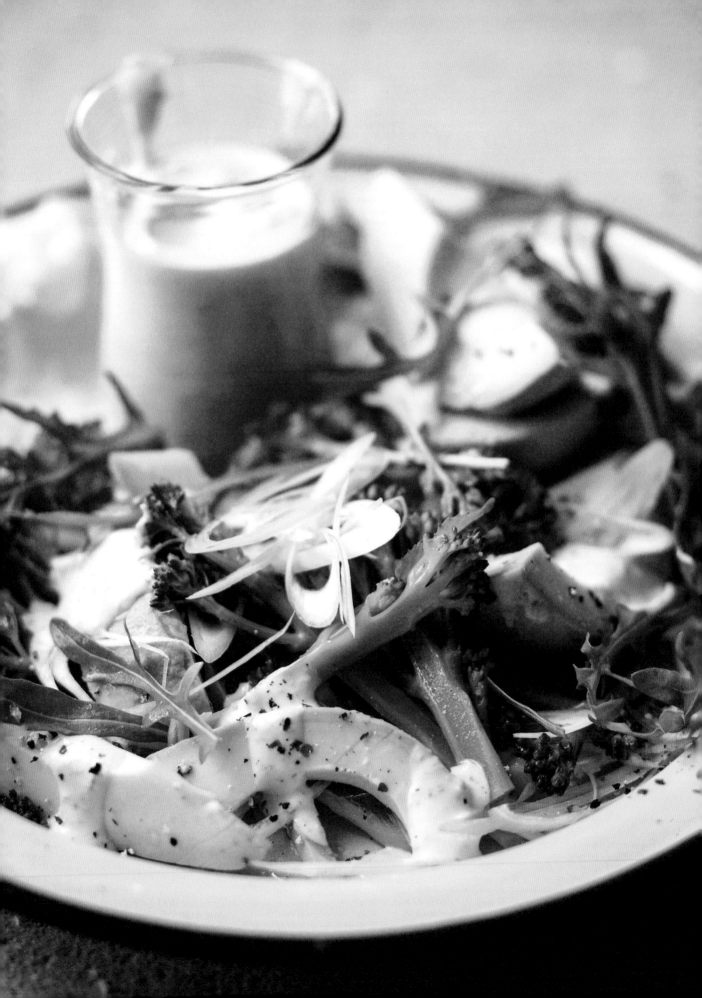

AVOCADO, SUGAR SNAP PEA AND MINT SALAD WITH POPPY SEED DRESSING

SERVES 2

FOR THE DRESSING

Juice of 1 lemon

2 tbsp red wine vinegar

1 tsp Dijon mustard

1 garlic clove, minced

4 tbsp poppy seeds, toasted

150 ml extra virgin olive oil

Salt and pepper

FOR THE SALAD

200 g sugar snap peas
or mangetouts

1 head butter lettuce,
washed and torn

1 large ripe avocado,
cut into chunks

1 bunch spring onions,
thinly sliced

1 large handful mint, picked
but not chopped

★ Make the dressing. Combine the lemon juice, vinegar, mustard, garlic and poppy seeds in a mixing bowl. While whisking continuously, pour in the olive oil until the dressing emulsifies. Season to taste.

★ Cut the sugar snaps in half lengthways on the diagonal.

★ Lay the lettuce leaves out on a platter. Layer with sugar snaps, avocado and spring onions. Cover with mint leaves and drizzle with the dressing.

★ Serve immediately.

Note: To give this salad more of a crunch, feel free to add any nut or seed from the green list (page 41).

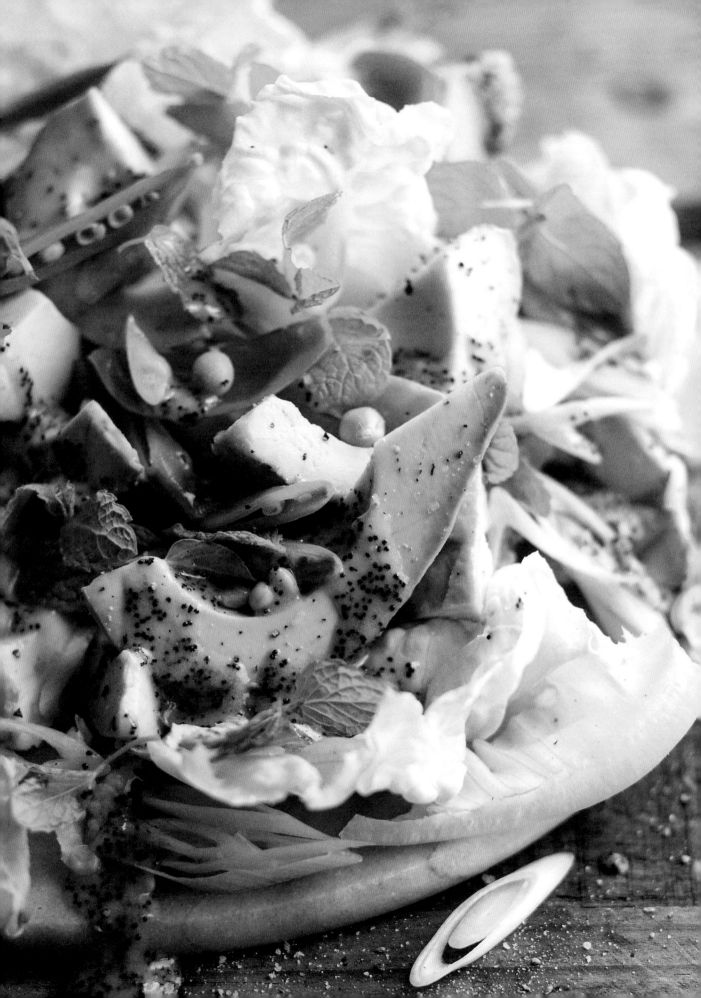

MARINATED TOMATO AND ANCHOVY SALAD

SERVES 4

These tomatoes go very well with pretty much anything. The anchovy and caper combo goes perfectly on top of a carpaccio or baked fish, but you can serve them just like this as a salad.

FOR THE DRESSING

Juice of 1 lemon

½ cup extra virgin olive oil

1 garlic clove, minced

1 huge bunch of flat-leaf parsley, washed

¼ cup capers, rinsed

3 tbsp anchovies (the best you can find)

FOR THE SALAD

150 g red cherry tomatoes, cut in half

150 g yellow cherry tomatoes, cut in half

6 large ripe tomatoes, cut into quarters

2 heads butter lettuce, washed

★ Make the dressing by combining all of the ingredients in a bowl or jug and blending them with a stick blender.

★ Place the tomatoes in a bowl and cover with the dressing. Leave them in the fridge, covered, for 12 hours or overnight.

★ Lay the lettuce leaves out on a platter and cover them with the tomatoes and the rest of the dressing.

Note: An amazing trick with this salad is to roast half of the tomatoes after they have been marinating. By roasting them you add a different texture to the salad and you also intensify all the flavours. I would highly recommend it.

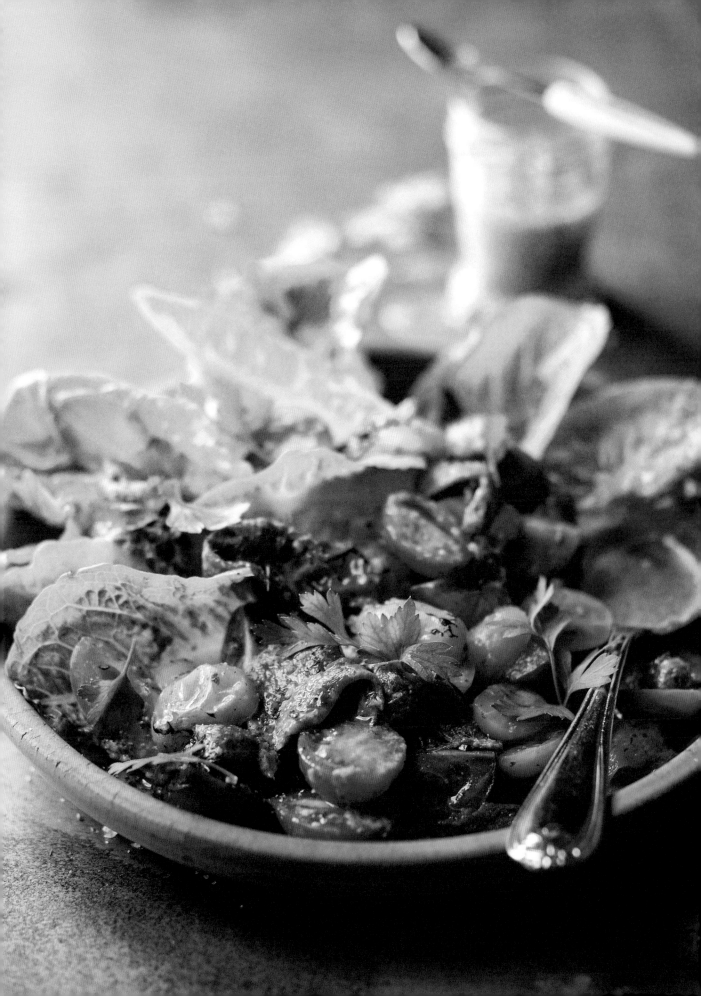

SPICED PUMPKIN AND GOATS' CHEESE, SUNFLOWER SEEDS AND CITRUS DRESSING

SERVES 4

Roasted pumpkin and any cheese is a match made in heaven. I prefer mixing it with stronger-flavoured cheeses like goats' cheese, blue cheese or hard cheeses such as pecorino and Parmesan, but it does stand up well to anything. Spices don't go particularly well with blue cheese or pecorino so I've gone with soft goats' cheese.

FOR THE DRESSING
Juice of 2 lemons
1 tbsp Dijon mustard
150 ml extra virgin olive oil
Salt and pepper

FOR THE SALAD
600 g pumpkin cubes
Coconut oil for roasting
1 tbsp ground cumin
1 tbsp ground coriander
1 tsp ground nutmeg
Salt and pepper
60 g rocket, washed
200 g creamy goats' cheese, broken into small chunks
¼ cup sunflower seeds

★ Preheat the oven to 180°C (Gas 4).

★ Toss the pumpkin in melted coconut oil, cumin, coriander, nutmeg and salt and pepper. Place on a tray and roast in the oven for about 45 minutes until nicely coloured on the edges.

★ Make the dressing. Combine the lemon juice and mustard in a mixing bowl and, while whisking continuously, pour in the olive oil until a dressing is formed. Season to taste.

★ Lay the rocket out on a platter and top with the pieces of pumpkin (once they've cooled).

Now add the chunks of goats' cheese, the sunflower seeds and finally, a liberal splash of dressing.

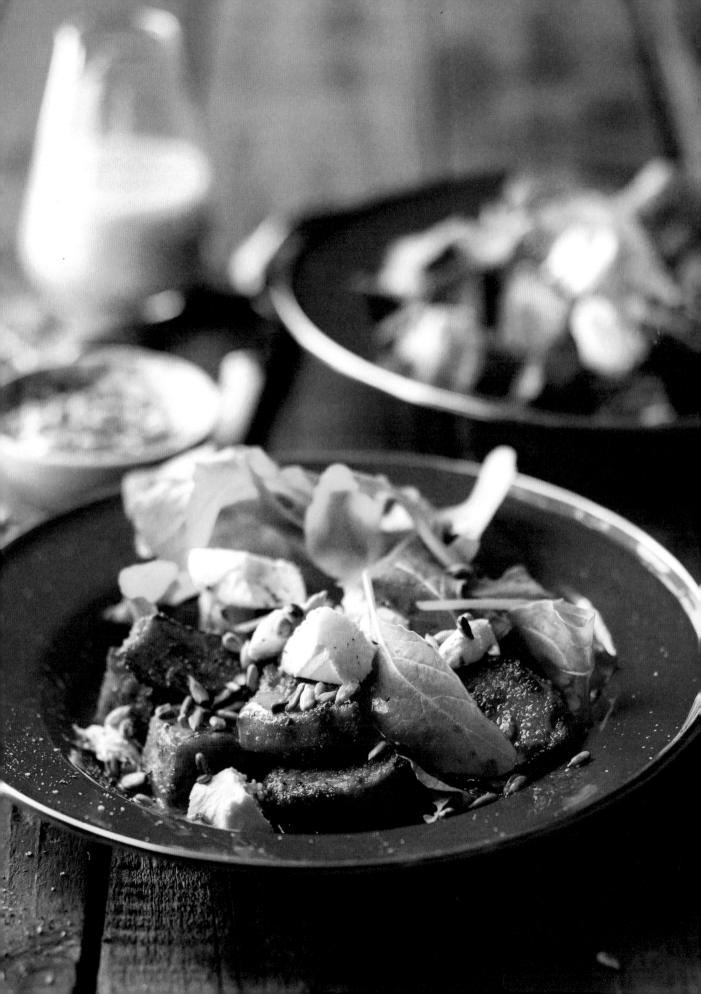

CHARRED HALLOUMI AND PEPPER SALAD

SERVES 4

FOR THE HALLOUMI

1 tsp cumin

1 tsp smoked paprika

1 tsp yellow mustard seeds

400 g halloumi, cut into
8 mm slices

½ cup olive oil

1 tsp dried thyme

1 tsp dried oregano

½ tsp salt

1 tsp ground black pepper

Basil sprigs to garnish

FOR THE PEPPER SALAD

2 large red peppers

2 large yellow peppers

100 g black olives

30 ml red wine vinegar

100 ml extra virgin olive oil

1 garlic clove, sliced

2 sprigs thyme

250 g cherry tomatoes,
roasted

60 g rocket

★ Put a griddle pan on the heat and get it smoking hot.

★ Combine the herbs, spices and seasoning with the olive oil and toss the halloumi in the mixture until it is well coated.

★ Grill each piece of cheese on the griddle pan for about 1 minute on each side. They should char on the outside but just about hold their shape. My advice would be to char these pieces in advance then place them on a tray. You can warm them in the oven minutes before you serve.

★ Make the salad. Char the peppers by placing them directly on the gas hob, whole, until they go pitch-black all over. Alternatively you can roast them in the oven or under the grill until blackened and soft.

★ Seal them in an airtight container and let them sweat until they cool (this helps separate the skin from the flesh).

★ Remove the peppers and use a knife to scrape the skin off the outside and the seeds from the inside of them.

★ Using your hands, shred the peppers into strips.

★ Add the peppers, olives, red wine vinegar, olive oil, garlic and thyme to a small saucepan. Bring to a simmer for about 5 minutes for the flavours to infuse and become absorbed by the peppers.

★ Lay the peppers, olives, cherry tomatoes, rocket and warm halloumi out on a platter.

★ Drizzle with the marinade from the saucepan and garnish with basil before serving.

Note: If you are doing a huge batch of these salads, you can assemble them, place them on an oven tray and warm them all under the grill just before you serve.

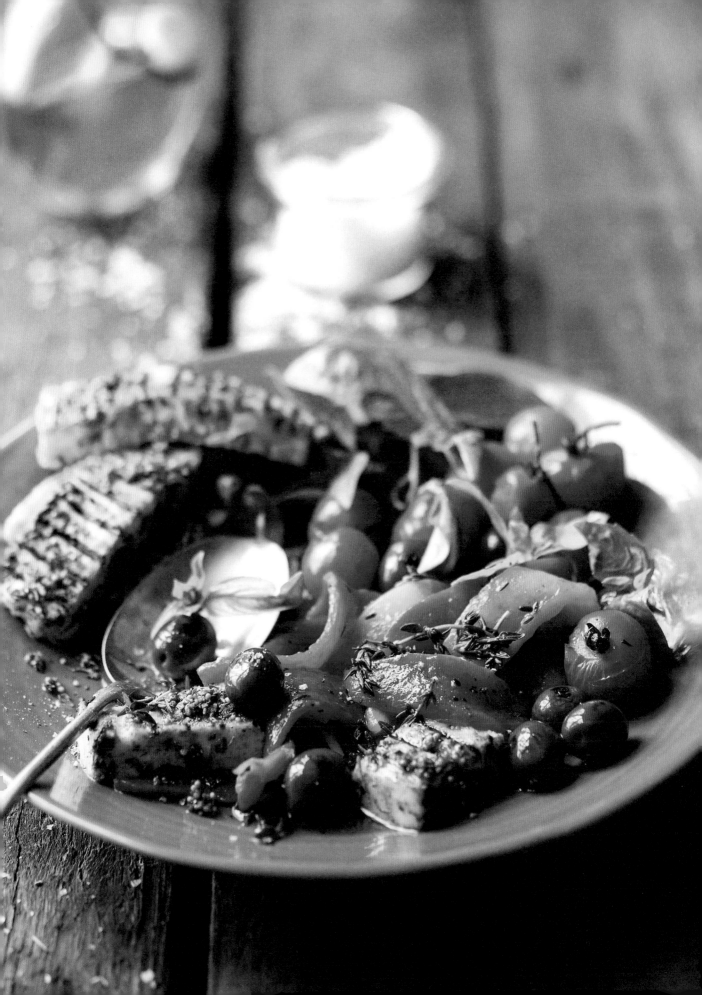

CHARRED AUBERGINES WITH PINE NUTS AND TAHINI

SERVES 4

This recipe uses aubergines but you could easily substitute courgettes using the same quantity.

FOR THE TAHINI SAUCE

4 tbsp tahini

1 garlic clove, crushed

Juice of 1 lemon

1 handful chives, finely chopped

FOR THE AUBERGINES

500 g aubergine, cut into wedges

3 garlic cloves, crushed

3 sprigs thyme, chopped

4 knobs butter

¼ cup toasted pine nuts

Salt and pepper

A good glug extra virgin olive oil

1 handful chopped flat-leaf parsley

★ Combine the tahini sauce in a small bowl. While whisking continuously, add drops of cold water one tablespoon at a time until you reach the consistency you like. Usually it will need about 100 ml water.

★ Preheat your oven to 220°C (Gas 7).

★ Get a griddle pan onto the heat at the highest temperature.

★ Grill each piece of aubergine on each side until they get charred lines and a good smoky flavour. (If the griddle pan is hot enough, you should not need oil for this, but feel free to brush the aubergines with a little olive oil before grilling.)

★ Once the aubergines are grilled, lay them down in a tray and dot with the garlic, thyme and butter. Season with salt and pepper.

★ Roast the aubergines in the oven for about 20 minutes or until dark brown. When they are cooked, remove from the oven and leave to cool.

★ Lay the aubergines out on a platter and drizzle liberally with the tahini dressing, then sprinkle with toasted pine nuts, freshly chopped parsley and good heavy glugs of extra virgin olive oil.

Note: apart from being a knock-your-socks-off item on the buffet table, these aubergines make for a great side served with lamb of any kind.

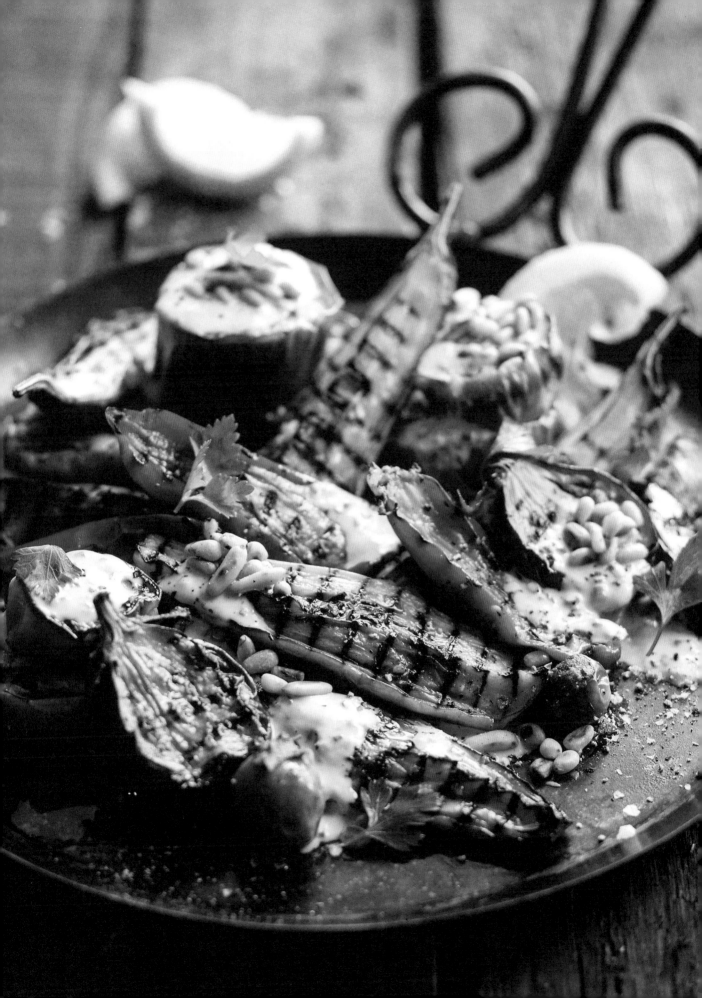

SCIENTIFIC JUSTIFICATION FOR A BANTING DIET

The comprehensive essay from Professor Tim Noakes

Most of us want to know what we should eat to optimize our health. The answer is perhaps rather simpler than we might think. It is found in the solution to the single most important question in the nutritional sciences. Which is: 'Why do all mammals not eat exactly the same foods?'

While there are obvious anatomical differences for example between giraffes, koala bears, panda bears, polar bears and lions, the commonalities in their shared biologies are much greater. Yet these similar mammals thrive by eating respectively acacia leaves, eucalyptus leaves, bamboo leaves and shoots, seals and grass- and shrub-eating game. So rigid are their specific dietary requirements that it requires little effort to discover which foods are best for these animals. We need simply to observe what they eat in the wild. Fed on any foods other than those that they naturally eat, all these animals will soon die.

The reason is quite simple: all creatures on planet earth must eat the foods for which they are designed; this design depends on the nature of their creation or evolution, according to your preference. This explains for example the advantage of the long neck of the giraffe (much better to access the acacia leaves that no other animal other than elephants can reach). Importantly acacia leaves cannot possibly provide all the myriad of nutrients required by the giraffe. So from where do these missing nutrients come? The answer has to be from the hundreds of trillions of bacteria that exist in the giraffe's massive intestine. Those specific bacteria are essential for the nutritional health of the giraffe. By providing some critical nutrients not present in the acacia plants, these life-sustaining bacteria insure not just the health of the giraffe but also the bacteria's own survival – a perfect symbiotic relationship. But change the giraffe's diet and the key bacteria in its gut will die followed shortly thereafter by the death of their host. Just as happens every few years on the Galapagos Islands as the changing water temperature causes a fatal reduction in the dominant seaweed on which the marine Iguana must survive. Iguana without the bacteria to metabolize this different seaweed will die. With stomachs full of undigested seaweed.

So it follows that if we want to establish which foods are best for modern humans, we need to discover which ones our early human ancestors ate before recent changes in our dietary options, especially those imposed by the Agricultural Revolution that began about 12,000 years ago.

Food choices before the Agricultural Revolution

Humans exhibit some unusual physical characteristics; these characteristics tell us much about our unique biology. For our height we have the longest legs of any mammals and surprisingly the greatest capacity to lose heat from our bodies through sweating. Modern-day elite but tiny human marathon runners weighing less than 60 kg can nevertheless sweat at rates of up to 3 litres/hr during competition. There has to be a biological reason why humans are designed to sweat so vigorously.

We also have (or at least we should have) thin waists and narrow hips that make it easier for us to run long distances without tiring. Humans also have a complex network of springs in our lower limbs that allow us to store energy in our muscles as our foot lands on the ground when running. That stored energy is then released as the muscles next contract propelling us forward with each stride. This reduces the energy cost of running, improving our efficiency and explaining in part why exercise is not an effective way to lose weight – humans are designed to use energy very efficiently and without waste when we exercise.

A similar network of springs surrounding our shoulders allows humans to throw balls with great velocity and accuracy, just as we once threw rocks and more recently spears.

All these findings suggest that humans are uniquely designed for efficient long distance running especially in the heat. Scientists now believe that early humans must gradually have realized that their design allowed them a competitive advantage. For through trial and error they would have discovered that over a period of hours they could effectively chase other non-sweating mammals until those animals became paralyzed by heat exhaustion.

At first, because it seems that males became the hunters, early males would have begun by catching the newly-born but defenceless offspring of the smaller antelope on the African plains – the impala, springbok and Thomson's gazelle – just as do modern baboons. As his expertise and courage grew he would have learned to observe where the leopard stashed its half-eaten prey. Then as a group many would

have discovered how to follow the cheetah and to chase it from its recently caught prey.

But the real advance occurred on an especially hot summer's day when a small band of early humans emboldened by the knowledge that their chief competitor, the lion, was lying somewhere in the shade incapacitated by the heat, set out to chase a much larger mammal like the Eland or the Gemsbok, to its exhaustion.

Over time the lean, linear, tall, long-legged, easy-striding modern human became the greatest endurance athlete on the planet. The only mammal, who because of an unmatched ability to sweat profusely from his entire body surface, is able to run without overheating in midday heat. And so to capture and devour the energy-rich bodies of the large non-sweating African antelope, on which humans were so utterly dependent at that time.

So it was that humans grew strong and clever on an energy-dense diet rich in fat and protein and provided by the bodies of savannah-dwelling antelope.

But early humans were not yet quite out of the woods, so to speak.

The Mossel Bay miracle?

Professor Curtis Morean from Arizona State University, USA believes there is a more recent but yet untold Southern Cape twist to this story. The problem with the popular explanation that the size of the human population has increased progressively over the years is that it does not explain why, compared to other species, humans show relatively little genetic variation. So little that many geneticists propose that all modern humans are descended from a small band of a few hundred surviving early humans who lived about 195,000 years ago either in East or South Africa. According to Morean's theory that small band survived the last modern Ice Age by discovering the only remaining site on the entire planet able to provide sufficient food to support their survival. And that natural Garden of Eden was, according to Professor Morean's research, the Southern Coast of Africa, specifically the region around Pinnacle Point near Mossel Bay.

There Morean contends modern humans lived in an area bounded on the South and East by the rich Indian Ocean teeming with fish and other marine life, and on the North and West by the land animals that humans had learned to hunt successfully. Easy access to a bounty of sea-foods was provided by a severe ice age that locked water at the North and South Poles lowering ocean levels and exposing the Continental Shelf off the Southern Cape coast for habitation and the gathering of especially marine food. And underground was the uniquely rich array of bulbs that comprise the Cape Floral Kingdom. The archaeological record suggests that during this period the human brain showed a quite dramatic increase in size almost certainly indicating that in their hardship this small band of humans had discovered a bounty of foods rich in fat and protein, ideal for optimum brain development.

If Morean is correct, it solves the problem of the foods with which early humans developed. We ate a diet rich in fat from fish and pasture-raised animals supplemented by a smattering of carbohydrates from tough fibrous underground bulbs. And those foods would have produced a specific intestinal bacterial flora that thrived on those natural foods and which in turn optimized human health.

Eventually the Ice Age ended and the progeny of the original humans spread from Africa crossing into Asia and Europe about 50,000 years ago. At first they would have continued their carnivorous ways searching for animals rich in protein and fat. In time this would have

taken them further north in search of those even fatter animals able to survive the harsh Northern winters.

And this reliance on animal foods produced a specific human metabolic profile best able to metabolize two of the major dietary macronutrients, fat and protein. But somewhat less well adapted to using the third macronutrient, carbohydrate.

Eating a diet rich in protein and fat but poor in carbohydrate produces a specific human metabolic profile – insulin (carbohydrate) resistance (IR).

Of the three macronutrients in our diet, only carbohydrate is completely non-essential for life. We cannot function properly for more than a few days without eating fat; without an adequate protein intake we develop protein-calorie malnutrition within a few months. But avoiding carbohydrate has no short- or long-term effects on humans, other than the (usually beneficial) effect of weight loss, especially in those who are the most overweight.

However humans cannot survive without a constant supply of glucose as glucose is an important fuel for the brain and certain other organs in fed (but not starved) humans. But this glucose can be produced by the liver from fat and protein and does not need to be ingested as carbohydrate in our diets. We call this process gluconeogenesis meaning the production of 'new glucose' (that is, glucose that is not ingested but produced from fat and protein).

The amount of glucose we need to produce each day by gluconeogenesis is kept small by our great human capacity to use fats as the preferred fuel for almost all our body's energy needs. The end result is that many, perhaps a majority of humans, exhibit a metabolic state known as insulin resistance, present to varying degrees from mild to severe in all of us, and in which we exhibit a wide variation in our capacities to metabolize ingested carbohydrate. It is this presence of varying degrees of insulin resistance (IR) in so many of us that, as we will describe, explains why our human health has deteriorated as we have moved increasingly to a diet comprising highly processed foods containing carbohydrate as the primary ingredient.

So this is the downside of our developmental history and the fact that at Pinnacle Point the only carbohydrates we ate were from the fibrous bulbs of the natural Cape Flora. For the carbohydrate in those bulbs is absorbed slowly and does not cause a marked increase in blood glucose and insulin concentrations. In modern terms those bulbs contain carbohydrates which have a low glycaemic index. Humans eating low glycaemic foods did not need to develop any special biological mechanisms to protect them from high blood glucose and insulin concentrations.

For we now know, not least because of the devastating consequences in those with uncontrolled type II diabetes mellitus (type 2 diabetes) that a high blood glucose concentration is very toxic for human tissues because glucose damages the structure of all proteins, the proper function of which are essential for our health. To minimize this effect, the only protective mechanism humans have developed is to secrete the hormone insulin whenever carbohydrate is ingested and the blood glucose concentration begins to rise. Under the action of insulin, ingested glucose is either used immediately as an energy fuel or it is stored in the liver and muscles. And any carbohydrate that cannot be so removed must be converted immediately into fat, first in the liver before being transported to the fat tissues for storage as fat. In order to maximize this use of carbohydrate, insulin also prevents fat from being used as a fuel. Hence insulin is the

hormone of both fat building and fat storage (by preventing its use as a fuel).

But the efficiency with which these processes occur in each of us is determined by the degree to which we are either IR or its opposite, insulin sensitive.

The degree of IR differs markedly in different humans and in different populations. In its most extreme form, IR is the key abnormality present in type 2 diabetes, the form of diabetes that occurs increasingly with older age in persons still able to produce some insulin. (The other less common form of type I diabetes, mellitus (T1DM), occurs in persons at a younger age, usually children, who lose their capacity to produce insulin as a result of irreversible damage to the insulin-secreting beta cells of the pancreas.) While the cause of the destruction of these pancreatic beta cells is still debated, the most recent theory is that in susceptible individuals it is caused by the development of the 'leaky gut' syndrome as a result of a diet high in wheat products. The 'leaky gut' then allows entry of bacterial proteins from the gut into the bloodstream. These proteins may then be mistaken as an invading infection and the body may respond with a full-on immune response. If any of the antibodies produced against the invading proteins should cross-react with proteins within the body – for example those found in the pancreatic beta cells – then the outcome will be the complete destruction of those cells leading to T1DM.

The tissues, liver and muscle especially of type 1 diabeties are not necessarily insulin-resistant, although they may be since there is likely to be a strong genetic predisposition to IR. Those with the most severe IR will develop severe obesity and type 2 diabetes at the youngest ages; those with mild IR may notice only that they struggle to control their weight and that their blood pressure tends to rise as does their fasting blood glucose and insulin concentrations as they pass beyond middle-age.

But perhaps more important is the idea that IR is the hidden metabolic abnormality underlying many of the chronic diseases currently reaching epidemic proportions in modern humans and which includes obesity, type 2 diabetes, high blood pressure, high blood cholesterol concentrations and heart disease (Figure 1).

Perhaps the reason why these diseases are now reaching epidemic proportions in all populations eating the modern American diet of highly processed, carbohydrate-rich foods is because those are the exact foods that people with IR are the least able to metabolize safely.

And it was this state of IR that best preserved us through those tough years at Pinnacle Point. But when we moved into Asia 50,000 years ago, trouble was on the horizon. For it was in Asia that humans were to make the first of their two catastrophic modern dietary blunders.

Paradise ends with the invention of agriculture – the first great modern human dietary disaster

Beginning about 13,000 years ago, humans living in Western Asia, also known as the Middle East, began to domesticate animals and to cultivate grasses, the ancestors of our modern cereals including wheat and barley. In this way cereals and grains were added to the human diet, reducing human reliance on hunting, fishing and gathering.

The exact reasons for this choice remain uncertain – some have suggested that the addictive nature of these grains on the human brain could have played a role. But this dietary revolution produced a dramatic reduction in human health. Compared to the skeletal remains of those who continued to follow a hunting existence, the bones of those who began to eat cereals and grains reveal a sorry tale of greatly impaired human health. And the clearest evidence of this can be found in the bodies of the Egyptian mummies.

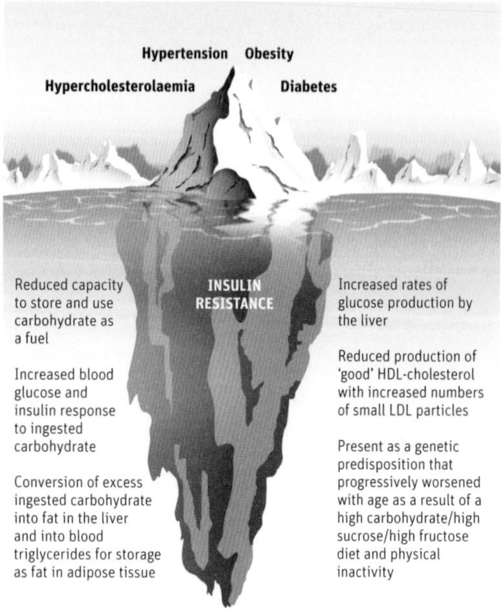

Hypertension   Obesity

Hypercholesterolaemia   Diabetes

INSULIN RESISTANCE

Reduced capacity to store and use carbohydrate as a fuel

Increased blood glucose and insulin response to ingested carbohydrate

Conversion of excess ingested carbohydrate into fat in the liver and into blood triglycerides for storage as fat in adipose tissue

Increased rates of glucose production by the liver

Reduced production of 'good' HDL-cholesterol with increased numbers of small LDL particles

Present as a genetic predisposition that progressively worsened with age as a result of a high carbohydrate/high sucrose/high fructose diet and physical inactivity

FIGURE 1: Diabetes, obesity, hypertension (high blood pressure) and hypercholesterolaemia are manifestations of a common underlying condition – insulin resistance (IR) – some of the biochemical features of which are shown in this figure.

The first experiment with the 'heart-healthy' low-fat, high-carbohydrate cereal-based diet: A story of widespread ill-health revealed in the mummified bodies of the Ancient Egyptians. Not only did we become sicker but we became smaller and fatter and life expectancy halved from an average of forty to twenty years.

The Egyptians living in the lush Nile Valley for the 3,000 years between 2,500 BC and 395 AD existed on a diet comprizing mainly carbohydrates, especially wheat and barley, which they baked into a flat whole-wheat bread. So great was their fondness for bread that Egyptian soldiers were known as 'the bread eaters'. Egyptian farmers also grew a wide variety of fruits and vegetables, including grapes, dates, melons, peaches, olives, nuts, apples, garlic, onions, peas, lettuce and cucumbers. The result was that the Egyptian diet of that period exactly matched that which would, after 1977, be promoted as the absolute epitome of modern, healthy eating.

In his book, *Protein Power*, Dr Michael Eades, MD describes what the Egyptians ate: '[The Egyptian] diet consisted primarily of bread, cereals, fresh fruit, vegetables, some fish and poultry, almost no red meat, olive oil instead of lard, and goat's milk for drinking and to make into cheese – a veritable [modern] nutritionist's nirvana.' If such is the ultimately healthy diet 'rich in all the foods believed to promote health and almost devoid of saturated fat and cholesterol [and refined sugar]' as we are now taught, then according to Eades, the 'ancient Egyptians should have lived forever or at least should have lived long, healthy lives and died of old age in their beds. But did they?'

The mummified bodies of the Ancient Egyptians bear mute testimony to the truth. From their decayed teeth and severely diseased gums to their obesity, widespread arterial disease and high blood pressure, the bodies of these mummies warn of the dangers of a cereal-based high-carbohydrate diet: 'So a picture begins to emerge of an Egyptian populace, rife with disabling dental problems, fat bellies, and crippling heart disease ... Sounds a lot like the afflictions of millions of people in America today, doesn't it? The Egyptians didn't eat much fat, had no refined carbohydrates ... and ate almost nothing but whole grains, fresh fruits and vegetables, and fish and fowl, yet were beset with all the same diseases that afflict modern man. Modern man, who is exhorted to eat loads of whole grains, fresh fruits, and vegetables, to prevent or reverse these diseases'. Eades concludes that this historical evidence might suggest that 'there are some real problems with the low-fat, high-carbohydrate diet'.

If only humans had learned from this natural experiment, we might have been spared the second great modern dietary disaster of 1977.

The second great modern human dietary disaster: The United States Senate Select Committee on Nutrition and Human Needs produces the 1977 *Dietary Goal for Americans (USDGA)*

Twelve thousand years later humans were ready for their second catastrophic dietary blunder. Sadly this one should never have occurred since it owes its existence purely to political and commercial factors and, as told by Nina Teicholz in her gripping book, *The Big Fat Surprise*, a distortion of science on an unprecedented and unimaginable scale. Its key effect was to spread the false gospel that the foods that humans had always eaten had, quite suddenly in the middle of the twentieth century, transformed into the direct cause of all our modern ill-health, most particularly to a rising incidence of heart disease that began after the end of the First World War (1918).

The false diet/heart hypothesis of Ancel Keys, PhD, introduces the 'plumbing theory' of how human heart disease develops

The theory that (saturated) fat in the diet raises the blood cholesterol concentration which then causes heart disease is known as the diet-heart/lipid hypothesis. Others call it the 'plumbing theory' of heart disease. It owes its existence principally to the missionary zeal of a single scientist, the American biochemist Ancel Keys, PhD. In 1953 Keys published a scientific paper in which he showed an apparent relationship between the amount of fat in the diet and the heart disease rates in six different countries (Figure 2). He concluded that this proved that by raising blood cholesterol concentrations, the fat in the diet clogs the arteries of the heart (the plumbing theory) and so must be the direct cause of heart disease.

But there were at least four problems with Keys' 'science' that continue to go unchallenged by those devoted to his plumbing theory.

First, he selected the data from only six of the twenty-two countries for which he had information. Data from those six countries provided the best visual representation of his theory as they fitted a perfect straight line.

Second, he failed to warn that the simple association of two observations does not prove that they are causally linked. That most men who suffer heart attacks are either bald or have greying hair or both does not prove that grey hair and balding causes heart disease any more than umbrellas cause rain. Causation can be proved only by randomized controlled clinical trials (RCTs) in which all variables except the one of special interest are held constant. Keys only ever reported observational studies; he did not undertake a single RCT to test this specific question as truly great scientists must do. For the goal of science is always to disprove that which we hold to be most obviously true. Science advances through disproof of our personal scientific biases. Not through continually 'proving' what we already believe to be self-evident and 'well established'.

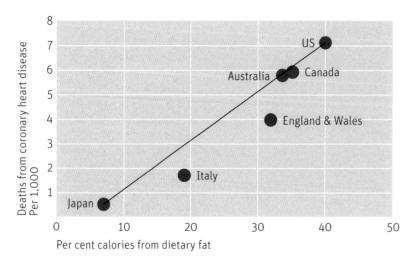

FIGURE 2: In 1952 Ancel Keys, PhD, published a paper apparently showing a strong linear relationship between the amount of fat ingested by the citizens of six different countries and the incidence of heart disease in those countries. This iconic figure was used as 'proof' of the still unproven theory that fat in the diet causes heart disease. This study shows an association between two variables. But associational studies can prove nothing.

Thus, in contrast to what many medical students and nutrition scientists in South Africa and elsewhere are taught, because he did not undertake RCTs, Keys could not ever prove the diet-heart hypothesis 'unequivocally'.

Third, Keys spent much of his life defending his theory against the criticism that any of a number of other confounding variables could explain, at least as well, the apparently causal relationship he preferred. For example the single greatest environmental change after the First World War, and which could conceivably be the sole important factor explaining the sudden rise in heart disease thereafter, was the growth in cigarette consumption after 1918 (Figure 3). But Keys was on a mission and so he ignored any possible contribution that other factors like smoking could have made to the suddenly rising heart disease rates after 1918.

Finally, Keys was not a clinician. He did not ever treat a single patient suffering from the disease about which he became the world's leading theorist. Sometimes a little practical knowledge can be helpful.

But Keys was not without critics, the chief of whom was Professor John Yudkin, then Professor of Nutrition and Dietetics at the University of London. Yudkin argued that differences in heart disease rates could as well be explained by differences in annual income between countries; that is, that growing levels of affluence were the real cause of the rising incidence of heart disease. Famously, he showed that the rising heart disease rate in the United Kingdom after the First World War was associated with the increasing number of radio and television licences owned by UK citizens. Clearly neither a television nor a radio licence can cause

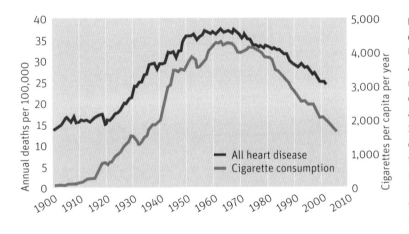

FIGURE 3: The annual number of deaths from heart disease in the United States began to rise shortly after the end of World War I. The rise and subsequent fall in heart disease deaths nicely tracks the rise and fall of cigarette consumption. Smoking is one of the most potent causes of heart disease so that these two events could be causally related. Instead, led by scientists like Ancel Keys, PhD, after 1953 the US decided to find a specific nutritional cause for the rise of heart disease, ignoring any potential role for changing smoking patterns in the US. Fat, especially saturated fat, was the chosen nutritional villain even though the consumption of saturated fat in the US has been falling since the early 1900s. But the consumption of sugar and polyunsaturated 'vegetable' oils has increased exponentially over the same time period.

'artery clogging'. Yudkin also showed a close relationship between dietary fat and sugar intakes in forty-one countries as well as a tight relationship between sugar intake and heart disease rates in the fifteen countries for which data were then available. So, he argued if countries with the highest saturated fat intakes also have the highest sugar intakes, how is it possible to choose between the saturated fat or the sugar as the 'cause' of their heart disease? Then in a series of research studies he showed that patients with disease of their arteries, including those supplying the heart, ate nearly twice as much sugar as did those without those diseases. Others subsequently confirmed an almost perfect relationship between the amount of sugar eaten in different countries and their respective rates of heart disease.

Thus already in the 1970s the evidence implicating sugar as a dietary factor associated with coronary heart disease was at least as strong as that incriminating dietary saturated fat.

But the definitive rebuttal to Keys' false doctrine was presented already in 1957 by two New York scientists, Drs Yerushalmy and Hilleboe. They analysed a wide range of possible associational relationships with heart disease from twenty-two countries, including the sixteen ignored by Keys concluding that: '... the evidence from twenty-two countries for which data are available indicates that the association between the percentage of fat calories available for consumption in the national diets and mortality from arteriosclerotic and degenerative heart disease is not valid; the association is specific neither for dietary fat nor for heart disease mortality. Clearly this tenuous association cannot serve as much support for the hypothesis which implicates fat as an etiologic factor in arteriosclerotic and degenerative heart disease.'

Today we know that the association between the percentage of saturated fat in the diet and

the incidence of heart disease in all European countries is inverse (Figure 4) – that is those countries with the highest percentage of saturated fat intakes like France and Switzerland have the lowest rates of heart disease whereas those with the lowest intakes of saturated fat have the highest rates. The Swiss are particularly interesting because they are among the longest-lived people in the world. Yet of all Europeans they have among the highest average blood cholesterol concentrations – the opposite of what Keys' doctrine would predict. Indeed there is no evidence that countries with high rates of heart disease have higher average blood cholesterol concentrations than those with lower rates of heart disease. In fact the evidence appears to be the opposite (Figures 5 and 6).

Furthermore, grouped analyses of all the published evidence shows that the amount of fat in the diet is unrelated to heart disease risk in individuals and that reducing dietary fat intake over many years does not change heart attack risk. But for those with IR, replacing fat in the diet with carbohydrate is unlikely to be a healthy choice. And even for the healthy, replacing saturated fat with polyunsaturated 'vegetable' oils, as promoted by the 1977 USDGA, cannot be healthy because it increases the intake of unhealthy omega-6 and trans-fats while reducing the intake of healthy omega-3 fats found in butter and other dairy produce from pasture-raised animals. Moreover, an increasing body of evidence suggests that the 'vegetable' oils may be linked to an increased risk for both heart disease and cancer.

Thus, were he alive today, Keys would be quite unable to produce any of the 'proof' that in 1957 he believed to be 'unequivocal'. In fact all the evidence should by now have finally buried the diet-heart 'plumbing' hypothesis for heart disease. That it has not is because of the wealth and influence of the pharmaceutical industry

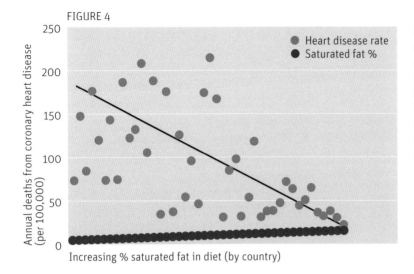

FIGURE 4

FIGURE 4: Annual deaths from coronary heart disease in European countries ranked (from left to right) by increasing percentge of saturated fat in the diet. Note that an increasing percentage of saturated fat in the diet is associated with reducing annual deaths from heart disease – the opposite of Ancel Keys's speculative theory.

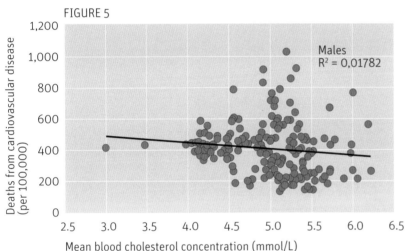

FIGURE 5

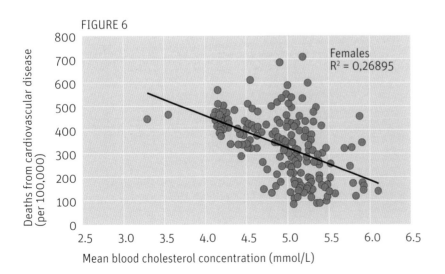

FIGURE 6

FIGURES 5 and 6: Cardiovascular disease death rates and mean blood cholesterol concentrations in 171 countries sampled by the World Health Organization. Figure 5 shows data for men; Figure 6 for women. Note that the relationship is inverse. That is, the higher the blood cholesterol concentrations, the lower the cardiovascular disease death rates. Total mortality showed exactly the same relationship, falling as a linear function of increasing blood cholesterol concentrations. The findings in Figures 4, 5 and 6 refute absolutely the diet/heart hypothesis of Ancel Keys.

on the medical profession and especially in determining what medical students are taught. Indeed, the modern 'science' of cardiology is crucially dependant on the continued support of the pharmaceutical industry. And this requires that the 'plumbing' theory of heart disease must be defended at all costs since without it there is no justification for the prescription of cholesterol-lowering statin drugs, a $40 billion a year enterprise.

But might these European data showing an inverse association between saturated fat in the diet and incidence of heart disease (Figure 4) support an opposite theory; specifically that saturated fat in the diet protects against heart disease?

Perhaps, but no credible scientist today would perpetuate Keys' cardinal error of claiming that association proves causation. If differences in heart disease rates between European countries are indeed due to dietary and not other factors, then perhaps they are due to differences in what people do not eat, rather than what they eat. These would include an increased consumption of especially sugar, high fructose corn syrup, cereals and grains and other refined carbohydrates, and vegetable oils in those countries with higher rates of heart disease. The increased consumption of any or all of these rather than a lesser intake of dietary saturated fat might then explain why those eating the least saturated fat are also the least healthy.

But the result is that today we know that there is no credible evidence linking heart disease with the amount of saturated fat in the diet. And anyone or any organization continuing to promote that incorrect information is guilty of misrepresenting what is now a firm body of disproof.

The real tragedy is that the removal of fat from the human diet, as advocated by Keys and his disciples, is very likely the single direct cause of the obesity (Figure 7) and diabetes epidemics that begin after 1980.

Which raises the question: 'Why did these twin epidemics begin in 1980? And not before, or after?'

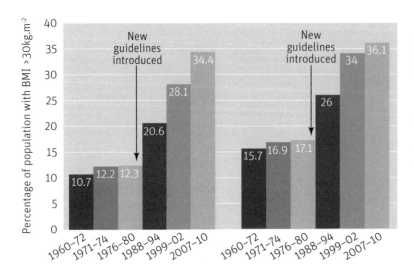

FIGURE 7: The rising incidence of obesity in the US begins in 1980, 3 years after publication of the 1977 USDGA which promoted the removal of fat from the diet and its replacement with carbohydrates (from http://www.cdc.gov/nchs/nhanes.htm). The graph on the left is for males, the graph on the right for females.

The industrialization of corn production in the United States after 1970

Just as Keys was formulating his false theory, political events were conspiring that would expedite the global expansion of his false diet-heart hypothesis. In 1972 US incumbent US President Richard Nixon was confronted with a losing and increasingly unpopular war in Vietnam, by rising food prices and by a disgruntled farming community. He appointed Earl Butz as Secretary of Agriculture with two orders: Bring down the price of food and increase the wealth of US farmers. Butz decided that the production of corn and soy on an industrial scale by farmers working as a huge conglomerate, receiving large state subsidies and planting every spare acre with grains was the solution to both 'problems'. His actions would have momentous effects on global health. Perhaps if there is one single person we can blame for the current obesity/diabetes epidemic, it is Secretary Butz (with help from 'Tricky' Dick Nixon).

For the industrialization of corn and soy production so achieved would be of little value if all the newly grown grains were not eaten, first by US citizens and their livestock and then by the rest of the world. But how to convince the world that grains and cereals are healthier than the foods high in protein and fat that all previous generations of healthy Americans had always eaten? Enter Senator George McGovern and his side-kick, vegetarian Nick Mottern.

The 1977 Dietary Goals for Americans (USDGA)

After a series of cursory interviews with selected scientists, in 1977 Senator George McGovern and his Senate Select Committee on Nutrition and Human Needs released the first Dietary Goals for Americans (USDGA). These novel guidelines driven by powerful commercial and political forces to insure the growth of US farming through the industrialization of wheat, corn and soy production were based entirely on Keys' unproven and subsequently disproven diet-heart hypothesis. These new guidelines mandated 'healthy' Americans to restrict their intake of especially saturated fats and cholesterol (in eggs) and instead to base their diets on at least eight to twelve servings of grains and cereals per day. These grains and cereals, foreign to all humans until as recently as 12,000 years, would replace the high-protein and fat foods like butter, lard, milk, cream, cheese, eggs and meat that until then had been the American staples. Instead those staples of human nutrition were relegated to the third tier of the soon-to-become ubiquitous Food Pyramid (Figure 8) that has dominated the teaching of human nutrition ever since.

These 1977 USDGA Guidelines, compiled by the vegetarian Nick Mottern, who had no formal training in nutrition science and who selected only the expert information that fitted his personal conviction, were criticized by Dr Philip Handler, then President of the National Science Academy (NSA). Handler posed the question: 'What right has the federal government to propose that the American people conduct a vast nutritional experiment, with themselves as subjects, on the strength of so very little evidence that it will do them any good?' He added: '... resolution of this dilemma turns on a value judgement. The dilemma so posed is not a scientific question; it is question of ethics, morals, politics. Those who argue either position strongly are expressing their values; they are not making scientific judgements'.

Similarly a leading cholesterol expert of the time, Professor Eric Ahrens, noted that: '... a trial of the low-fat diet recommended by the McGovern Committee and the American Heart Association has never been carried out. It seems that the proponents of this dietary change are willing to advocate an untested diet to the nation on the basis of suggestive evidence obtained in tests of a *different* diet. This illogic is presumably justified by the belief that benefits will be obtained, vis-à-vis CHD prevention, by *any* diet that causes a reduction in plasma lipid [cholesterol] levels'.

No matter. The Food Pyramid and these untested guidelines were soon promoted and supported by a range of other US Government agencies, not least the National Institutes of Health (NIH) which began to focus increasing amounts of its research budget to provide the definitive 'proof' that persons who followed the 1977 USDGA would become immune especially to heart disease, obesity and diabetes. Note that the function of research organizations like the NIH should be to support research that aims to disprove not to prove existing 'truths'.

Unfortunately the three major research projects funded by the NIH over the past 40 years – the Framingham Study, the Multiple Risk Factor Intervention Trial (MRFIT) study and the $700 million Women's Health Initiative Randomized Controlled Dietary Modification Trial (WHIRCDMT) – all failed spectacularly to 'prove' that this dietary change produced significant health benefits. The exposure of this failure is fully described by Nina Teicholz in *The Big Fat Surprise*. The most interesting of these studies is perhaps the WHIRCDMT, the goal of which was to determine whether post-menopausal women who adopted a 'heart-healthy' low-fat diet, high in vegetables, fruits and grains, reduced their risk of developing cardiovascular disease (CVD). The trial substantially favoured the intervention group who also received an intensive nutritional and behaviour education program not offered to the control group. Of course this diet is

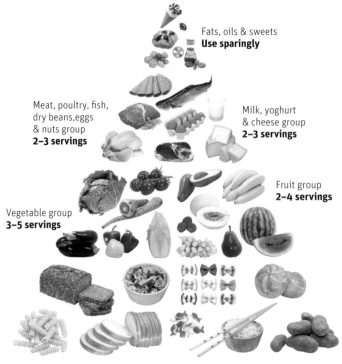

Fats, oils & sweets
Use sparingly

Meat, poultry, fish, dry beans,eggs & nuts group
2–3 servings

Milk, yoghurt & cheese group
2–3 servings

Fruit group
2–4 servings

Vegetable group
3–5 servings

Bread, cereal, rice & pasta **6–11 servings**

FIGURE 8: The Food Pyramid promoted by the 1977 USDGA. The pyramid relegates the foods traditionally eaten to the third tier, replacing them with 6–11 servings a day of foods that were first introduced to humans only 12,000 years ago and which were followed immediately by a reduction in human health, best exemplified by the diseased bodies of the Ancient Egyptian mummies.

exactly that which made the Ancient Egyptians so ill. Had the NIH scientists understood the archaeological record, they could have saved their masters $700 million. Imagine if these scientists had chosen rather to study the diet that healthy Americans had favoured for the three centuries before the heart disease 'epidemic' began after 1918 (Figure 3).

The authors' conclusion after more than eight years of study was that: '... a reduced total fat intake and increased intake of vegetables, fruits, and grains did not significantly reduce the risk of coronary heart disease [CHD], stroke, or CVD in postmenopausal women and achieved only modest effects on CVD risk factors'. In fact, this hugely expensive and carefully conducted study made a number of inconvenient discoveries that the authors glossed over and which have since been conveniently forgotten.

First, post-menopausal women with heart disease at the start of the trial had a 26 per cent increased risk of developing heart disease during the trial if they adopted the 'healthy' low-fat diet compared to women who continued to eat the traditional unhealthy diet with a higher fat content. Second, women who were either

lean or middle-aged at the start of the trial were more likely to gain weight during the trial if they ate the low-fat diet. Third, the healthiest women were more likely to develop diabetes if they reduced the fat in their diet whereas the condition of those with established diabetes was also more likely to worsen if they did the same.

If the 'healthy' low-fat diet ever had a chance to prove its success, this $700 million trial was the best chance. But it failed. Yet this is not ever acknowledged by those who continue to promote the now disproven 'low-fat is healthy' dogma.

Within five years of the widespread adoption of these new dietary guidelines, global rates of diabetes and obesity increased explosively, especially in the United States. The damage caused by the adoption of the 1977 USDGA began to appear quickly. By 1994 American men had increased their daily energy intakes by 7 per cent and American women by 22 per cent (Figure 9). Beginning after 1980 there was also an immediate (8 per cent in men and 9 per cent in women) increase in the rates of obesity in the USA within the same fourteen years (Figure 7), perfectly matching this increased intake of calories especially from carbohydrate.

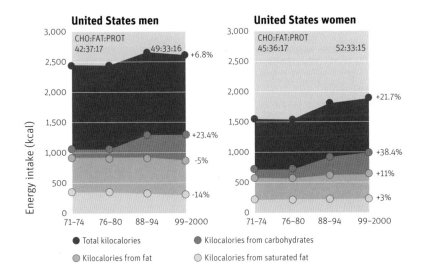

FIGURE 9: Nutritional intake data (total kilocalories; kilocalories from carbohydrates, fat and saturated fat) for United States men (left) and women (right). Note that intakes of total kilocalories and kilocalories from carbohydrate, fat and saturated fat remained stable from 1971–80. After 1980, however, total kilocalories and kilocalories from carbohydrates rose markedly. The USDGA promoting increased carbohydrate intakes were introduced in 1977. (From Hite et al. 2010)

Any increased intake of carbohydrates by those with IR would be more than enough to explain the simultaneous rise in global obesity and diabetes rates.

This tight linkage by both time and plausible biological mechanism between the increased carbohydrate intake promoted by the 1977 USDGA and the rising incidence of obesity and diabetes after 1980 is the final evidence we need to prove that these dietary guidelines have had a catastrophic effect on global health.

The third catastrophic modern human dietary disaster: genetically modified foods

Modern carbohydrate food sources differ substantially from those tough fibrous Cape Floral bulbs on which the pioneering humans survived at Pinnacle Point 200,000 years ago. Today especially the sweetened fruits and carbohydrate-rich vegetables that we eat bear no resemblance to those less sweet and poorly digested foods that existed in nature at the time of the Agricultural Revolution. The result is that modern fruits and vegetables have a higher usable carbohydrate content that is rapidly assimilated within the human body. This causes a steep rise in blood glucose concentrations, setting off a steep increase in blood insulin concentrations, especially in those with more marked levels of IR.

In addition the fruits that were available at Pinnacle Point were seasonal, unlike the modern provision of fruits all year round.

In the last few decades the cereal and grains that constitute the six to eleven servings that we are encouraged to eat daily (Figure 8), have undergone substantial genetic modification, not to improve our health but to increase their profitability. As a result, a typical slice of modern bread raises the blood glucose and insulin concentrations as quickly as does the same weight of glucose. By raising our blood glucose and insulin concentrations so rapidly and repeatedly modern bread is killing us just as surely as did the cereals and grains favoured by the Ancient Egyptians.

Re-establishing balance: The growth of low-carbohydrate eating with reversion to our ancestral eating patterns

Chefs, it seems, know best when it comes to what we should be eating. The first person to suggest that a high-carbohydrate diet promotes weight gain even in healthy humans was French gastronome Jean Anthelme Brillat-Savarin. Already in 1825 Brillat-Savarin had concluded that: 'All animals that live on farinaceous [starch-rich] substances become fat; man obeys the common law' so that as 'farinaceous food produces fat in man as well as in animals, it may be concluded that abstinence from farinaceous substances tends to diminish embonpoint [plumpness]'.

Brillat-Savarin's thinking had perhaps been influenced by his escape from Paris to New York in 1793 to evade the Christian persecution. He was surprised by the plumpness of the New Yorkers and wondered if this was due to either their Dutch heritage or the 'extraordinary amount of pastries, pies, sweets and corn-products eaten'.

But it was not Brillat-Savarin who would be immortalized for this insight that carbohydrates, not fats, make humans fat. Rather that honour belongs to an unlikely Englishman, the formerly chubby William Banting.

In 1862 Banting, a well-connected and prosperous London undertaker, self-published the first edition of his fourteen-page *Letter on Corpulence, Addressed to the Public,* in which he described his lifelong battle with obesity and its apparently miraculous cure following the adoption of a novel eating plan prescribed by his ENT surgeon, Mr William Harvey. Banting had consulted Harvey to find a cure for his growing deafness. Harvey concluded that Banting's problem was his obesity that was causing pressure on the nerves in his ears. Not aware of Brillat-Savarin's conclusion, Harvey had decided independently that a diet containing 'farinaceous' foods was fattening so that logically the avoidance of starchy foods was the key to the treatment of obesity.

Banting's *Letter on Corpulence* sparked unprecedented public interest in the role of a low-carbohydrate diet for the treatment of obesity. But Harvey's dietary advice was initially shunned by the medical community as he was unable to explain why his treatment was effective. In time he proposed that the inclusion of generous amounts of protein, not the avoidance of carbohydrate, produced this dramatic weight loss. As a result he modified the original diet to include more protein and less fat, a change which Banting considered inferior to the original (higher-fat) version. Instead a German physician, Dr Wilhelm Ebstein, became the principal advocate of the original low-carbohydrate, high-fat (LCHF) moderate protein version of the Harvey/Banting diet.

In his monograph published in 1884, Ebstein wrote the following: 'This property of fat to produce satiety more rapidly, to diminish the craving for food and abate the feeling of thirst, facilitates to an extraordinary degree the introduction of the modified diet . . . . The permission to enjoy certain things, always of course in moderation, as for instance salmon, pâté de foie gras and suchlike delicacies reconciles the corpulent gourmet to his other sacrifices (which) consist in the exclusion of carbohydrates. Sugar, sweets of all kinds,

potatoes in every form I forbid unconditionally. The quantity of bread is limited at most to 3 to 3½ oz. a day, and of vegetables I allow asparagus, spinach, the various kinds of cabbage and especially the leguminous, whose value as conveyers of albumen (protein) . . . is known to few. Of meats I exclude none, and the fat in the flesh I do not wish to be avoided, but on the contrary sought after. I permit bacon fat, fat roast pork and mutton, kidney fat, and when no other fat is at hand I recommend marrow to be added to the soup. I allow the sauces as well as the vegetables to be made juicy, as did Hippocrates, only for his sesame oil I substitute butter . . . In spite of all this it would be little to the point to say that I treat the corpulent with fat, whereas I simply vindicate the full claims to which fat is entitled as an article of food' (pp. 43–44).

Acceptance of the Banting/Ebstein diet spread throughout Europe and was initially promoted in the United States (US) by Dr William Osler, Professor of Medicine at Johns Hopkins University in Baltimore, Maryland, USA. Osler is an iconic figure in global medicine as he wrote the world's first medical textbook evaluating how effective the array of medical treatments available in 1892 were. His conclusion: Not very.

Yet in his iconic textbook Osler prescribed the high-fat version of the Banting/Ebstein diet as *the* treatment for obesity. So in the 1892 words of perhaps the most famous medical practitioner of all time we find:

'Many plans are now advised for the reduction of fat, the most important of which are those of Banting, Ebstein and Oertel. In the Banting (Harvey) method the amount of food is reduced, the liquids are restricted, and the fats and carbohydrates excluded'.

'Ebstein recommends the use of fat and the rapid exclusion of the carbohydrates ... Farinaceous and

all starchy foods should be reduced to a minimum. Sugar should be entirely prohibited. A moderate amount of fats, for the reasons given by Ebstein, should be allowed' (p. 1,020).

The point is that the very first diet books ever published assumed it self-evident that carbohydrates cause obesity and that carbohydrate restriction is the only treatment for obesity. Hence one must conclude that diets for weight loss that are not based on carbohydrate restriction can legitimately be labelled as 'fad diets' since they are different from those adopted as effective by the medical profession, including its most famous clinician of the 1900s, if not of all time.

The low-carbohydrate diet was also promoted in the US by the writings of archaeologist Vilhjalmur Stefansson, who had lived with the Arctic Inuit for more than a decade sharing their exclusive fat/protein diet. On his return to the US, Stefansson wrote a book entitled *Not by Bread Alone* and became the subject of a year-long laboratory trial during which he avoided all carbohydrates including vegetables and fruits. Despite the researchers' certainty that he would likely die from scurvy, Stefansson quickly lost 2 kg in the first week and a further 2 kg within the first month, remaining in perfect health for the duration of the trial. His experiences inspired a long lineage of low-carbohydrate diets, which he labelled consecutively the Eskimo Diet, the Friendly Arctic Diet, the Blake Donaldson Diet, the Alfred W. Pennington Diet, the Du Pont Diet and the Holiday Diet. The popularly maligned Atkins Diet (1972) is just one of the most recent examples in this 150-year lineage of low-carbohydrate diets that begins with Harvey and Banting. In fact there are now probably close to 100 books that have been written about the Low-Carbohydrate High-Fat (LCHF) diet, with most appearing in the past five to seven years.

Unquestionably it was Dr Robert Atkins' *Diet Revolution*, published in 1972, that has been the most influential of all these books. Unfortunately for Atkins his book appeared at the exact moment that President Nixon, facing re-election, had decided to increase the wealth of US farmers and bring down the price of food by industrializing the production of grain, especially maize and soy. Clearly there was no place for an upstart New York doctor to be telling Americans that they should eat the foods that Americans had always eaten – meat rather than maize, saturated fat and not grains.

If Atkins made one substantial error it was that he failed to undertake clinical studies on the more than 60,000 patients it is estimated that he treated for obesity and related conditions at his New York clinic over the four decades that ended with his death in 2003. Only shortly before his death, perhaps after he had contracted a form of heart disease caused by a viral infection, did he encourage and fund a group of scientists led by Drs Jeff Volek, Stephen Phinney and Eric Westman to study the effects of his diet on various health parameters. This work has established that the Atkins Diet consistently outperforms the diet based on the 1977 USDGA in all parameters measured.

Unfortunately this information has yet to become part of the mainstream teaching in either medicine or the nutritional sciences. An excellent source of this information can be found on the website of Authority Nutrition, in which the first twenty-three studies showing the superiority of the LCHF over the HCLF Diet is reviewed: http://authoritynutrition.com/23-studies-on-low-carb-and-low-fat-diets. More recently, the twenty-fourth such study has been published with the same finding (Bazzano et al., 2014). It is perhaps time for more to appreciate that the science supporting the value of the LCHF eating plan is strong, while that favouring the low-fat diet is in rapid retreat (Teicholz, 2014).

South African experience with the LCHF Diet: Prof Tim Noakes

As described in my book, *Challenging Beliefs*, in December 2010 I embarked on a personal experiment, adopting the Banting Diet. The results were so spectacular that I decided to speak about them publicly, beginning about a year later in December 2011. This soon became something of a national issue and many in both the medical and dietetics professions were less than happy with my successful weight loss following my dietary conversion. Some wondered if I had the necessary qualifications to propound on nutrition; others stated publicly that I had finally lost my senses. A number of leading professional organizations in South Africa used the public media to warn all South Africans that the 'Tim Noakes diet' is dangerous and will damage their health. They were warned that they should most definitely not ever consider changing their 1977 USDGA 'heart-healthy' diet for the dangerous, artery-clogging 'Tim Noakes' option.

Nevertheless many thousands of South Africans ignored this advice, choosing rather to experiment along the lines of the simple dietary advice I had posted on the internet. In time some of those who had experienced successful outcomes wrote to thank me for solving their weight and health problems that the 'time honoured' (but unproven) conventional advice had failed to cure. Included in those communications were 127 from subjects who reported the exact amount of weight each had lost. Many included additional health information. An analysis of this information was subsequently published in the *South African Medical Journal*.

Remarkable weight loss reported by the 127 subjects

The 127 subjects reported a total weight loss of 1,900 kg. Remarkably, the average weight loss (-15 kg) far exceeds that usually reported in expensive clinical trials typically involving the HCLF Diet under intensive medical supervision and costing many millions of dollars. The data from this observational study establish what well-motivated subjects can achieve in the real world even without supervision, suggesting the LCHF intervention is indeed a remarkably potent weight-loss and health-promoting intervention.

By comparison, a combined analysis of nearly 60,000 subjects participating in a number of different studies of the low-calorie HCLF Diet reported an average weight loss of only -1.6 kg. Another self-help study of the HCLF produced an average weight loss of only -1.3 kg at one year and -0.2 kg at two years. This evidence confirms that in those who really wish to lose weight by sticking to a few simple rules, the Banting Diet is far more effective than the HCLF. I now finally understand why this is so. Crucially, I would never have reached this insight had I not myself experimented with the Banting Eating Plan.

The role of sloth and gluttony as a cause of obesity in these subjects

The popular energy balance model of human obesity discussed subsequently predicts that the overweight chose that outcome because they are consciously slothful and gluttonous. The experience of these 127 subjects shows that many presumed slothful and gluttonous persons have a remarkable capacity to lose weight when they adopt the Banting Eating Plan and at the same time avoid addictive food choices.

Thus most of the 127 subjects had each tried repeatedly and unsuccessfully to lose weight on a 'healthy' HCLF Diet. As a result those who were the most overweight had each essentially relinquished any hope of ever again being a reasonable body weight. Billy Tosh's remarkable experience of losing 83 kg in twenty-eight weeks (Case 1) is described below. Brian Berkman, who lost 73 kg on the LCHF, sought refuge in bariatric surgery from which only his poor state of health saved him. Dr Gerhard Schoonbee, a fifty-seven-year-old general practitioner who suffered from type 2 diabetes, high blood pressure, 'high' blood cholesterol concentration, an abnormal heart rhythm (atrial fibrillation) and sleep apnoea, each treated with a different medication under specialist care, had informed his wife that he would be dead by age sixty-five. On the 'heart-healthy' HCLF he had been continuously hungry and unable to sustain any significant weight loss nor reverse any of his five potentially fatal medical conditions. Yet on the LCHF he quickly lost 25 kg and cured all his conditions so that he no longer requires the use of any medication. A twenty-three-year-old mother who developed (gestational) diabetes during her first pregnancy had tried numerous different weight-loss methods, all of which had failed as she would eventually 'cheat' and regain any lost weight. She had never been informed of the addictive nature of her food choices yet as soon as she adopted Banting she lost 45 kg in ten months.

Despite significant training volumes, Simon Gear, a marathon runner, could not prevent a progressive weight gain with age. He thought that running nine marathons in nine weeks would produce a miraculous weight loss; instead his weight increased by 3 kg. After adopting Banting his weight loss was greatest when he exercised the least. More interestingly, Simon reduced his finishing time in a 56-km South African ultramarathon by nearly three hours and his finishing position by over 7,400 places, finishing in 208th position.

But if sloth and gluttony alone cause obesity, then none of these subjects should have been able to reverse their obesity since such character defects are presumably immutable. That 127 subjects reported large weight losses confirms that this remarkable weight-loss response to the LCHF is not restricted to a few 'biologically abnormal' human variants. Crucially a large number of respondents spontaneously indicated that they had never been able to lose weight and keep it off as effortlessly as with the LCHF eating plan. What might explain this unexpected response?

Banting acts by reducing or removing hunger

Through my personal experience on the Banting Diet I discovered for myself that the key determinant of whether a particular eating plan will produce successful long-term weight loss is, unquestionably, the extent to which the new diet reduces hunger and as a direct consequence caloric intake. Twenty-seven of the 127 subjects spontaneously reported that their symptoms of hunger were dramatically reduced or absent on Banting. This was most obvious in the two star cases, Billy Tosh and Brian Berkman, who lost respectively 83 and 73 kg while Banting without hunger despite eating only a fraction of the calories they had previously needed to satisfy their food cravings (and addictions).

So the key to the remarkable efficacy of the Banting Diet appears to be its capacity to produce satiation despite a reduced energy intake. In contrast, the hypocaloric HCLF Diet usually fails because it produces the opposite – increased hunger. As Professor John Yudkin noted in 1958 'the high fat-diet is in fact a low-calorie diet'.

Indeed it was Professor Yudkin who first documented what I have termed the 'Yudkin paradox'. In 1970 Professor Yudkin and his colleague, Dr Anne Stock, reported a study in which they switched the diets of eleven subjects from a typical 'heart-healthy' 2,330 calorie/day HCLF Diet providing 216 g/day of carbohydrate (57 per cent of total calories) to one in which they could eat as much as they liked, provided they restricted their carbohydrate intake to less than 70 g/day. Remarkably, when eating to hunger on this Banting Diet the eleven subjects spontaneously reduced their total calorie intake to 1,560 calories/day, a reduction of 33 per cent (770 calories). Analysis also found that total fat and protein intakes did not change when converting from the HCLF to the Banting Eating Plan. Thus the only change was an ~150 g/day reduction in daily carbohydrate intake.

Stock and Yudkin also reported: 'In conformity with our experience with this diet during the last 15 years, none of our subjects complained of hunger or any other ill effects; on the other hand, several volunteered statements to the effect that they had increased feelings of well-being and decreased lassitude'.

So the paradox. Despite eating fewer calories subjects were less hungry and more energetic. But our every instinct tells us that this cannot be true. For we presume that hunger is satiated by eating more calories and especially more fat. But in this case hunger was satisfied even though fewer calories and only the same amount of fat were eaten.

So how can we explain this? The answer has to be that it is the removal of carbohydrate from the diet that reduces hunger – not the provision of more calories from fat. Thus carbohydrates stimulate appetite – they do not reduce appetite.

Surprisingly the evidence that the Banting is either 'at least as effective' or more effective than the hypocaloric HCLF for producing effective weight loss is thoroughly documented

in the scientific literature but appears to be consistently underplayed by those committed to promoting the 'heart-healthy' HCLF Diet for health and weight control.

Other health benefits: Banting cures some cases of type 2 diabetes, high blood pressure and 'elevated' blood cholesterol concentrations

Following adoption of Banting, fourteen subjects with type 2 diabetes reported that they no longer require medication to control their abnormal blood glucose concentrations, indicating that Banting 'cured' their type 2 diabetes, an outcome which years of expensive pharmacological intervention had been unable to achieve in some. A further eight with type 1 diabetes or type 2 diabetes were able to reduce their use of diabetic medication following adoption of the Banting Eating Plan.

The finding that Banting improves glucose control more effectively than does the HCLF Diet in those with impaired carbohydrate metabolism is established although seldom acknowledged. Instead South African patients with either type of diabetes are usually encouraged to eat diets in which carbohydrate provides at least 40 per cent of daily calories and more than 130 g/day. It is not proven that this is the best advice.

Historically, before the discovery of insulin patients with type 1 diabetes were managed on very high-fat carbohydrate-restricted diets since 'carbohydrates taken in the food are of no use to the body and must be removed by the kidneys thereby entailing polydipsia, polyuria, pruritus and renal disease'.

Eight of the 127 subjects reported that the adoption of Banting cured their high blood pressure (hypertension); another seven were able to reduce their anti-hypertensive medication after adopting this eating plan.

Another five subjects reported that their 'elevated' blood cholesterol concentrations, for which they were receiving cholesterol-lowering drugs, had normalized so that they no longer needed to use such medication.

This suggests that in addition to its remarkable effects in morbid obesity, Banting should be considered as a treatment option to cure type 2 diabetes, hypertension and 'elevated' blood cholesterol concentrations in some people without the need for life-long medication. This is important since modern pharmaceutical agents can cure none of these conditions.

But what these findings really prove is that obesity, type 2 diabetes, hypertension and 'elevated' blood cholesterol concentrations all have a common cause, which is a high-carbohydrate diet in those with IR (Figure 1). Understanding this explains why the LCHF can cure all these conditions.

Indeed, if these 'diseases' can be reversed in many by simply removing carbohydrate from the diet, are they really 'diseases'? This is the question explored by Jeffrey S. Bland in his book, *The Disease Delusion*. Bland suggests that these conditions are not diseases so much as they are abnormal biological responses to an abnormal insult, in this case a high-carbohydrate diet (in those with insulin resistance – Figure 1).

If this conclusion is correct, it poses an enormous challenge for the modern medical treatment paradigm which is based on the idea that foreign chemicals, in the form of patented designer drugs, are the sole therapeutic option for all the chronic diseases that afflict modern humans. But if these diseases are no more than a temporary diet-induced derangement in our metabolism, that can be reversed by returning to the foods that our ancestors ate, then do we

really need all those patented medicines?

In 1939 Dr Weston Price published the first edition of his classic book describing the health of traditional peoples eating their traditional foods, *Nutrition and Physical Degeneration*. He noted the absence of almost all of the chronic diseases that now plague twenty-first century humans. Is it too large a leap of faith to postulate that these modern diseases are caused by the modern foods that we are now eating?

So, how did the 1977 USDGA produce the obesity/diabetes epidemic?

By reducing 'artery-clogging saturated fats' overstuffed with calories, the USDGA was meant to prevent both heart disease and obesity. But as so often happens when theories are accepted on the basis of incomplete evidence, there is the probability that unintended consequences will result. The epidemic of obesity and diabetes that began after 1980 is a classic example. But how do we explain it?

The role of the brain's appestat in the regulation of human body weight

Any explanation of why humans have grown so fat quite recently must explain two irrefutable facts. First, that for almost all of our existence, humans have been lean. This tells us that the natural state of humans (like all non-hibernating wild animals except perhaps the elephant and the hippopotamus) is to be lean. Staying lean for all that time happened even though we did not have any conscious idea of what and how much we should eat each day to stay lean and healthy.

Instead we simply responded to the normal biological cues that accurately regulate our energy (food) intake so that it matches precisely

– to the final calorie – the amount of energy we need to sustain our daily physical activity and the integrity of our bodies.

This process is known as the homeostatic control of body weight through the precise matching of energy intake and energy expenditure. Some liken this control to the action of an appestat in the brain that regulates our appetite so that we are always just hungry enough to eat the exact number of calories that we need each day.

It follows that since humans have grown increasingly fat after 1980, then the cause must be damage to the appestat that kept us lean in the past. If we understand what has damaged the appestat, we understand what is causing the modern obesity epidemic.

An important clue is that the increase in obesity (Figure 7) occurred immediately after humans began to eat more carbohydrates (Figure 9) and processed foods than ever before. That we may also have become less active is irrelevant since a properly functioning appestat simply reduces hunger and the desire to eat in exact proportion to the reduction in energy expenditure. In this way we do not grow fat on the days that we do not exercise – we simply eat less that day and so maintain our weight constant.

Similarly, if we eat less than we should on any particular day or if we eat less for prolonged periods, the brain ensures that we also exercise less to conserve those calories. But the human brain does not do the opposite: if we eat too much because of our addictive food choices, the brain does not force us to exercise more and so to burn off those excess calories. In fact the opposite happens – as they gain weight, the obese become less inclined to exercise. Thus some suggest that a disinclination to exercise is not a cause of obesity, but rather the result of the metabolic abnormalities present in the obese.

As the predicted reduction in daily physical activity since 1980 is the equivalent of about 100 calories/day – about the number of calories present in half a slice of bread – a properly functioning appestat would have had no difficulty reducing our daily food intake by the equivalent of half a slice of bread in order to prevent the obesity epidemic after 1980. Instead, the obesity epidemic is the singular proof that something in our environment has damaged the proper functioning of the appestat beginning after 1980.

Since it is much easier to overeat calories in food than to under-expend calories in physical activity so the most probable explanation is that the appestat was damaged by either (i) the increased intake of dietary carbohydrates following the direction of the USDGA to remove fat from the diet after 1977 or (ii) the increased intake of processed foods since 1980. Or a combination of both. (This does not exclude other factors playing a role but they would be complimentary, not directly causal.)

But how do the experts – the biologists and nutritional scientists – explain the sudden onset of the obesity epidemic after 1980? The answer is that most use the Energy Balance Model of Obesity as the basis for their explanation.

The Energy Balance Model of Obesity

This model of human weight control was first promoted in the early 1900s by the German diabetologist Carl von Noorden. He proposed that obesity is due simply to the ingestion of too many calories regardless of whether they originate from fats, carbohydrates, proteins or alcohol. This is best termed the Energy Balance Model of Obesity. An absolute acceptance of this model as the sole explanation for obesity soon gripped the world and lives on as the dominant global explanation. It is the reason why we are told that the sole way to lose weight is to ingest fewer calories, especially less fat, and to exercise more. The problem with this model is that it is brain-less. It includes no role for the brain in the development or subsequent management of obesity.

So according to this model we must regain control of our errant appestats by consciously matching the (reduced) number of calories we must eat each day with the increased number of calories we need to expend in physical activity. The fact that for the entire human history until 1980 the appestat has worked perfectly without requiring any conscious input is conveniently ignored by adherents of this calorie-counting model of weight control. So too is the fact that we can measure accurately the balance between energy intake and expenditure to about 500 calories/day whereas a mismatch of just 10 calories per day will produce obesity over a few years. In fact the only practical measure of calorie balance is our daily weight. If it is stable, our daily energy intake exactly matches our daily energy expenditure. Of that we can be certain.

A key requirement for this calorie-counting model of weight regulation is that we must be able to control our food intake on the basis of conscious regulators – in other words we can consciously choose to be the weight that we are. As a result if we gain weight it is simply because we have become slothful and gluttonous – we actively choose to do too little exercise and to eat too much. In a word, we lack discipline and motivation.

So, according to this model (Figure 10) the cause for the global obesity epidemic is really quite simple – it is the result of a massive, global failure of human willpower that began with that generation of humans born after 1980. So, if this is cause, then the solution is also simple. We must regain our resolve; we must correct our suddenly wrong energy balances. By counting

our calories, by controlling our portion sizes and by removing fat from our diets, we will again become lean. According to this logic a reduced-calorie, high-carbohydrate, low-fat (HCLF) diet of the kind favoured by the Ancient Egyptians will be the most effective weight-loss option.

Naturally it is easy to find evidence to support our bias. So we note that the obese are always stuffing their faces and never exercising. And each successive generation is becoming less active and eating more. So the energy balance model is obviously the correct explanation for what we see daily. (What we fail to note is the nature of the foods that the obese eat.)

A key problem with this explanation is that it has proved to be of essentially no practical value. Telling the obese that they are slothful, gluttonous and lacking in willpower and resolve and putting them on intensive exercise training programs while forcing them to eat a starvation diet (without addressing the composition of that diet) is utterly unhelpful. It is the equivalent of telling an alcoholic that his problem is that he drinks too much alcohol. He already knows that, but this information has yet to save the life of a single alcoholic. Essentially the same applies to the obese. Telling the obese that they eat too much and exercise too little has not reversed the obesity epidemic. Not even stalled it. In fact it has probably accelerated it.

We know this because those who try to lose weight according to this HCLF approach show an impressive average weight loss of about 1.5 kg despite their best efforts and highest levels of motivation. And when they fail to sustain even that small weight loss we conclude that this simply proves what we already knew: that the obese are unmotivated and undisciplined. And so we blame the victims for their predicament. Worse, we conclude that obesity is the result of a human character flaw and is incurable. Only the lean are strong-willed; all the rest are unworthy of our efforts. Or our understanding.

But the fundamental unrecognized problem with the energy balance model is that it is brainless – it ignores any potential role for the human brain in regulating both energy intake and energy expenditure. It ignores the role of the appestat that for all but the last three decades of human history has been absolutely precise in directing exactly how much we need to eat each day to keep our bodies at a stable weight.

To reverse the obesity epidemic we have to understand that *obesity is a disease of the brain*. Unless we fix the appestat we cannot reverse the obesity epidemic.

So if this model has failed so abysmally, are there any others that might be a better option?

The hormonal (insulin) lipophilic (fat-loving) model of obesity

This model (Figure 11) is fundamentally different from the energy balance model since it offers a reasonable explanation of why people ingest too many calories and so become, and remain, obese. The model foretells that hormones and especially the fat-building hormone, insulin, are crucial drivers of weight gain (although it acknowledges that without an excessive caloric intake, there can be no obesity). The model

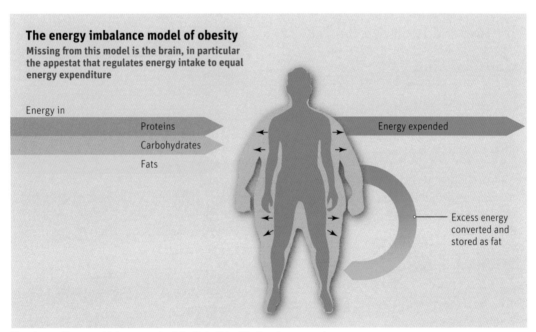

The energy imbalance model of obesity
Missing from this model is the brain, in particular the appestat that regulates energy intake to equal energy expenditure

Energy in

Proteins

Carbohydrates

Fats

Energy expended

Excess energy converted and stored as fat

Based on a diagram which appeared originally in *Scientific American* magazine

FIGURE 10: The British/American energy imbalance model proposes that obesity results from the intake of a greater number of calories from any combination of proteins, carbohydrates and fats than are expended in daily activities. As a result, the excess food energy is stored as fat. This model, which became popular after World War II, has dominated research and teaching in obesity since 1980; the precise period during which obesity has become a global pandemic. The model is wrong because, while it explains *how* obesity occurs, it gives no indication as to *why*. It fails to include the role of the brain and especially the appestat in controlling how much an individual eats (by determining levels of hunger and satiety) and how physically active he or she is.

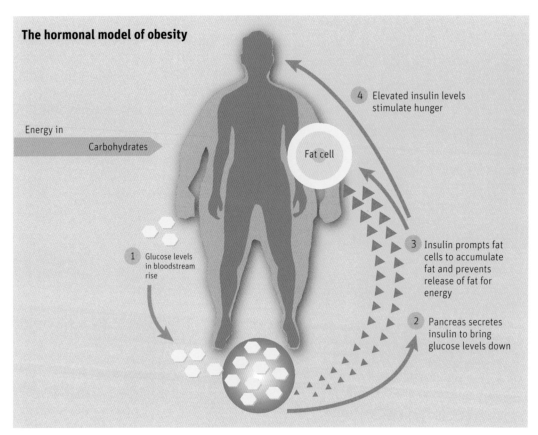

The hormonal model of obesity

Energy in

Carbohydrates

Fat cell

4 Elevated insulin levels stimulate hunger

1 Glucose levels in bloodstream rise

3 Insulin prompts fat cells to accumulate fat and prevents release of fat for energy

2 Pancreas secretes insulin to bring glucose levels down

Based on a diagram which appeared originally in *Scientific American* magazine

FIGURE 11: The (Austro-German) hormonal model of obesity was popular until the end of World War II when it was replaced by the British/American energy imbalance model. This model proposes that carbohydrates are uniquely fattening because they cause blood glucose concentrations to rise. In response the pancreas secretes insulin, which both lowers the blood glucose concentration but also drives the excess carbohydrate into fat in the liver and fat cells.

Hence insulin is known as the 'fat-building hormone'. Even at low blood insulin concentrations, insulin also prevents the release of fat from the fat cells. Thus insulin both builds fat and prevents the use of fat as an energy fuel. Ingested carbohydrate also stimulate hunger, in part because elevated insulin concentrations reduce the satiating effect of the hormone leptin from acting on the brain to reduce hunger – the condition known as leptin resistance.

also predicts that while all calories may be the same when measured outside the body, when ingested, calories from carbohydrate, fat and protein act quite differently in a complex organism like the human body. And calories from carbohydrate are uniquely obesogenic (obesity causing) for three different but complementary reasons.

First, carbohydrates stimulate the appetite and encourage the overconsumption of calories; that is calories from carbohydrate act differently on the appestat than do calories from fat and protein. Second, calories from carbohydrate cause increasing secretion of the fat-building hormone, insulin, that specifically stores as fat any excess calories ingested as carbohydrate. In addition, calories from fat require an input of (wasted) energy before they can be stored or metabolized within the body whereas carbohydrates do not. As a result calories from carbohydrate are not the same as calories from fat.

This hormonal theory of obesity has its origins in the first half of the twentieth century when German-speaking scientists realized that persons with early onset (type 1) diabetes start to lose weight the instant their pancreas fails to produce enough insulin (causing diabetes). Thus it was realized that 'a functioning pancreas is essential for the fattening process'. They also noted that fat accumulated in specific 'lipophilic' areas of the body, more readily in the obese than in the lean. In addition: 'Like a malignant tumour or like the foetus, the uterus or the breasts of a pregnant woman, the abnormal lipophilic tissue seizes on foodstuffs, even in the case of undernutrition. It maintains its stock, and may increase it independent of the requirements of the organism. A sort of anarchy exists; the adipose tissue lives for itself and does not fit into the precisely regulated management of the whole organism'.

Those ideas continue to be well recognized in modern textbooks of human physiology although its relevance has perhaps escaped the attention of medical practitioners and most nutritional scientists. Thus: 'Insulin not only promotes fat storage but it also restrains fat mobilization' and 'Lipogenesis [fat storage] is high in the fed state and following carbohydrate administration, whereas it is suppressed by fasting, high-fat diets, or insulin deficiency, such as in uncontrolled diabetes'.

Indeed, in the textbook from which I learned my physiology – perhaps the most famous such textbook in the world – the following is written: 'It will become apparent that insulin secretion is associated with energy abundance. That is, where there is great abundance of energy-giving foods in the diet, especially excess amounts of carbohydrate, insulin is secreted in great quantities. In turn, the insulin plays an important role in storing the excess energy. In the case of carbohydrates, it causes them to be stored as glycogen mainly in the liver and muscles. Also, all the excess carbohydrates that cannot be stored as glycogen are converted under the stimulus of insulin into fats and stored in the adipose tissue' (Guyton and Hall, 2006). There described is the mechanism by which obesity develops in response to the (over-) ingestion of carbohydrates.

So, although that is what most medical students in many English-speaking countries are taught, somehow we all forget the lesson. Especially when we are also taught that the one nutrient that does not cause insulin secretion – fat – is exactly the nutrient we should never eat.

Unfortunately the defeat of Germany in World War II and the adoption of English as the universal scientific language buried this theory until it was recently recovered through the remarkable writings of New York science writer Gary Taubes. Taubes's two recent books

Good Calories, Bad Calories and *Why We Get Fat and What to Do About It* are perhaps the single greatest reason for the growing academic interest in the insulin theory of obesity and the rise of the LCHF Eating Plan as the potential solution for obesity. The key benefit of the LCHF is that being low in carbohydrate, it stimulates neither appetite nor excessive insulin secretion.

The past decade has seen a dramatic increase in the volume of science published on the effects of the Banting Diet for weight loss, reversal of risk factors for heart disease and for improving athletic performance, most especially in those with insulin resistance. Some of the key studies have been provided by Drs Jeff Volek, PhD and Stephen Phinney, MD, whose ground-breaking work is summarized in their books, *The Art and Science of Low Carbohydrate Living* and *The Art and Science of Low Carbohydrate Performance*. It was these scientists who were the first to be funded by the late Dr Robert Atkins, MD, whose low-carbohydrate diet bears his name and who is the man considered by many to be the father of the modern low-carbohydrate movement.

As we will discuss subsequently, recent analyses indeed show that the Banting is more effective than the HCLF in reducing excess body weight and in reversing ALL the established risk factors for heart disease. Since this conflicts absolutely with conventional teaching it is not (yet) easily accepted.

Summary

So, in summary, the evidence is absolute. The singular and direct cause of the epidemic of obesity and diabetes that began in the first generation born after 1977 was the adoption of the scientifically-unproven 1977 USDGA that encouraged all the world's people to adopt a low-fat, high-carbohydrate diet. This also predicts that each succeeding generation since 1977 will be successively heavier. The biology of this effect is the following:

In the first place weight gain cannot occur without the ingestion of more calories than are needed by the body. In this sense the energy balance model of obesity is correct. But the point is that the over-ingestion of calories cannot occur if the brain appestat is functioning properly as it did in the majority of humans until 1980.

The appestat of the obese must fail because it is especially susceptible to the appetite-stimulating effects of high-carbohydrate foods, especially those found in modern processed foods that are designed with the single goal that they are also highly addictive. It is those addictive foods that, like a malignant cancer, have invaded the human food chain in the past thirty years.

So, we can conclude that the brain appestat of the obese is especially fragile and easily misled by too much carbohydrate, especially when present in highly addictive foodstuffs. Thus to reverse the obesity epidemic we have to understand that obesity is principally a disease of the brain that is induced by the addictive nature of the highly processed, sugar-drenched food-like substances that pass as our modern foods.

Next, we have the problem of too many IR humans.

Eating too many grams of carbohydrate each day will cause weight gain and perhaps even obesity, even in those who are not IR. But according to the hormonal (insulin) model of obesity, weight gain will occur much more easily in those who have an impaired capacity to metabolize carbohydrate because their tissues are IR. Thus in those with IR, carbohydrates are especially obesogenic because every time carbohydrates are eaten, they cause an exaggerated secretion of insulin which directs the excess ingested calories to be stored as fat. In addition the carbohydrates specifically cause the overconsumption of calories, not only because they fail to satisfy appetite (as they are usually eaten in foods that are not nutrient dense) but because they actively drive hunger.

Here is the step-wise sequence of how the promotion of a 'heart-healthy' high-carbohydrate diet must inevitably lead to obesity and diabetes in populations that include a sizeable proportion of individuals with appestats oversensitive to carbohydrates and addictive foods and bodies with varying degrees of IR.

HOW A HIGH-CARBOHYDRATE DIET OF ADDICTIVE FOODS MUST CAUSE AN OBESITY AND DIABETES EPIDEMIC IN HUMAN POPULATIONS WITH FRAGILE APPESTATS AND VARYING DEGREES OF IR

Early humans refined their biology in a low-carbohydrate environment and only occasionally ate rapidly assimilated carbohydrates (which cause blood glucose and insulin concentrations to rise rapidly, especially in those with IR)

Dr Morean's theory that humans were nearly wiped out as a species and survived only because of the fortuitous presence of the Continental Shelf off the Southern Cape coast helps explain why modern humans are so poorly adapted to eat a diet full of highly refined and easily absorbed carbohydrates. For at Pinnacle Point early humans enjoyed the bounty of the protein- and fat-rich seafoods harvested with little effort and to which the only added carbohydrate came from the tough, fibrous bulbs of the Cape Flora. On this diet we did not need to develop biochemical defences against sudden increases in blood glucose and insulin concentrations.

We now know that the blood concentrations of both glucose and insulin must be kept as low as possible as both cause long-term detrimental effects in humans. The long-term damage that occurs in insulin resistance is due to the effect of persistently elevated blood insulin, glucose and glucagon concentrations on many different organs. A key action of insulin is rapidly to lower the blood glucose concentration to limit that damage. But if insulin is persistently elevated, as occurs in those with insulin resistance eating a high-carbohydrate diet, the insulin adds to the glucose-induced damage by acting on those tissues that still retain their insulin-sensitivity.

According to the 'Father of Insulin Resistance' Dr Gerald Reaven, MD of Stanford University, persistently high insulin concentrations cause all of the following (Reaven, 2012):

★ Weight gain (insulin action on the appestat producing leptin resistance that interferes with the sensations of satiety)

★ Atherogenic dyslipidemia (comprising elevated blood triglyceride and small dense LDL-cholesterol concentrations and reduced HDL-cholesterol concentrations)

★ Visceral adiposity (insulin action on adipose cells)

★ Endothelial dysfunction

★ Hypertension (insulin action stimulating the sympathetic nervous system)

★ Hyperuricemia

★ Systemic inflammation

★ Mitochondrial dysfunction

★ Impaired exercise performance

Moreover, insulin is now considered to be an added factor explaining the increased risk for cancer, ageing and dementia in those habitually eating high-carbohydrate diets.

The key action of insulin in the obese with IR unable to burn much carbohydrate as a fuel is to remove the glucose from the bloodstream and convert it into fat in the liver. But insulin – the fat-building hormone – also prevents the body from burning that fat as a fuel. So all the extra dietary carbohydrate becomes locked up in the body's fat cells and under the influence of insulin cannot be accessed as a fuel. It simply remains locked within the fat cells.

By dietary fat elevates neither the blood glucose nor the blood insulin concentrations. Protein too has a much smaller effect on insulin secretion than does carbohydrate.

Humans do not have any essential requirement for dietary carbohydrate

Humans cannot survive unless they include fat and protein in their diets. But there is absolutely no requirement for carbohydrate so that humans can survive indefinitely without ingesting any carbohydrate. In fact carbohydrate serves only two functions in humans – it must either be burned as an energy fuel or stored as fat or carbohydrate (the latter is much reduced in the insulin resistant). There is no other option. Unlike fats and protein, carbohydrates cannot be used to build any of the body's structures.

This means that the grams of carbohydrate ingested each day must either be used every twenty-four hours as a fuel or they must be stored either as fat in the fat tissues or as glycogen in the muscles and liver. Persons with IR have a reduced capacity to burn carbohydrate as a fuel both during exercise and when at rest, or to store it as glycogen. As a result when they eat a carbohydrate-rich diet, those with IR will store most of the excess carbohydrate as fat, even if they perform prodigious amounts of exercise (in an attempt to burn off the excess carbohydrate). Some even argue that storing carbohydrate as fat is the way the human body is designed to cope with a toxic chemical (glucose), which until the Agricultural Revolution was not a major component of the human diet.

Thus the paradox: The single macronutrient, carbohydrate, which has established detrimental effects on our bodies and which for the human body has no dietary requirement is the one elevated to the status of a super-health food by the 1977 USDGA.

Humans differ in the ease with which they will gain weight when exposed to a high-carbohydrate diet

A large body of scientific evidence shows that IR, a hereditary predisposition present in a large percentage of humans, is the root cause of especially obesity, diabetes, heart disease, high blood cholesterol concentrations and high blood pressure (Figure 1). According to this model, those with the highest degree of IR will develop the visible manifestations of this condition, such as the onset of obesity and type 2 diabetes, at the youngest ages.

The prevalence of IR increases with age so that in the US it is claimed that 75 per cent of adults over the age of sixty-five have IR. The rising incidence with age is linked to, among others, a lifelong high-carbohydrate intake, especially of refined carbohydrates and fructose in sugar and high fructose corn syrup, and decreased levels of physical activity.

While there is a large body of evidence supporting this theory, it is not taught in medical schools or in schools of nutrition for the reason that it offers a quite different treatment method than that currently favoured by conventional medicine. For the conventional teaching is that obesity, diabetes, heart disease, high blood cholesterol concentrations and high blood pressure are each separate diseases treated by separate specialists using different treatments according to the current medical model which believes that there is a single cure for each medical disease and that cure is a specific pharmacological agent, or drug. The intellectual basis for the practice of modern medicine and nutrition is undermined if all these diseases share a singular cause, IR, and a common therapy which is not the prescription of a specific drug but simply the restriction of the amount of carbohydrates in the diet.

This is the unfortunate explanation as to why Banting is so threatening to so many who presently earn their living in either medicine or nutrition.

The important practical point is the following: Persons with IR are never able to eat much carbohydrate if they wish to optimize their health. Insulin resistance does not improve with age – it is more likely to grow progressively worse. In the words of Dr Robert Atkins, MD: 'As long as you look upon being *off* your [low-carbohydrate] diet as part of your future plans, you will *never* solve your weight problem. This can only happen when you accept the reality that if you have a weight problem, you must stay on a diet for life.'

His message is simply the following: those with IR can only ever control their weight especially, but also their health, if they restrict the number of grams of carbohydrate they eat each day. This requirement is for life. So the Banting 'diet' that rapidly improves their health cannot ever be abandoned. It must be followed for life. It must mature from a 'diet' to a life-long eating plan.

Hunger is the ultimate determinant of the overconsumption of calories that leads to obesity. So the key feature of the obese is that they are always hungry

Obesity cannot occur without an overconsumption of calories. And the chief driver of the overconsumption of calories is, not surprisingly, hunger. Thus to understand the obesity epidemic ultimately comes down to understanding why the collective global appestat has failed since 1980. This requires that we understand what drives hunger and how this was warped by the 1977 USDGA.

Hunger is regulated by two factors in the foods

we eat – the first is their bulk and the second their nutrient density. Bulky foods fill the stomach and produce a rapid satiation whereas nutrient-dense foods turn off hunger for much longer. Importantly, carbohydrates and protein/fat foods act quite differently on both these directors of our hunger.

So, carbohydrate-rich foods like pasta, potatoes, cereals, bread and many vegetables – the food encouraged by the 1977 USDGA – are bulky and when eaten, they quickly fill the stomach, producing a more immediate satiation. But because these foods are not nutrient dense, their satiating effect passes quite quickly and hunger usually returns within an hour or two. That is why a pasta meal is never quite enough.

As a result most people eating high-carbohydrate diets must eat every three hours as they are continually hungry. In this way repeated ingestion of high-carbohydrate foods encourages a high-calorie intake even in those who try to eat less by denying their hunger.

In contrast and in ways that we do not yet fully understand, foods with high nutrient density satiate hunger over much longer periods – six to twelve hours. The easiest way to show this is to compare the time of day when one's hunger returns after eating either a 'healthy' sugar- and cereal-based high-carbohydrate breakfast with added fruit or eggs, bacon and low-carbohydrate dairy products. Hunger usually returns within three hours after the 'healthy' breakfast whereas it may be early afternoon before one again begins to think about food after a low-carbohydrate breakfast.

So, the key discovery when persons change from eating carbohydrate-rich but nutrient-poor foods to nutrient-dense 'real' foods of the kind that we have always eaten is that within a few days hunger disappears. No longer must we eat every three hours. Instead with hunger satiated we are freed to eat only when circumstances are right – that is when the right foods are available. Not when our hunger forces us to eat addictive, highly processed foods of convenience which may satiate hunger for a short time but do not prevent the return of an exaggerated hunger a few hours later.

In this way nutrient-poor, carbohydrate-rich foods promote frequent eating and the chronic overconsumption of calories as clearly documented in the United States since 1977 (Figure 7).

Addictive foods produce continual hunger and so are the key drivers of the obesity/diabetes epidemic

Investigative reporter Michael Moss has provided a game-changing book entitled *Salt Sugar Fat: How the Food Giants Hooked Us*. The book contains two key revelations.

The first is that Moss describes how the manufacturers of processed foods use a special testing method to identify the 'bliss point' which is the 'precise amount of sugar or fat or salt that will send consumers over the moon' (p. xxv). So, processed foods are engineered specifically to maximize their addictive potential, to ensure that we will always 'crave' these fake foods. And so to ensure that the consumer keeps eating these 'irresistible' foods addictively without concern for the predictable long-term negative health consequences.

To compound the problem, the industry uses other 'devious moves: lowering one bad boy ingredient like fat while quietly adding more sugar to keep people hooked' (p. xxvi). So, the ultimate marketing trick – labelling unhealthy high-sugar processed foods as 'healthy low-fat' options. And the whole world fell for the scam. How could we have been so compliant? And so naively stupid?

Moss's second revelation is the one with which he begins his book – a meeting in Minneapolis in April 1999 when the eleven men who control the US processed food industry met to hear Michael Mudd, vice-president of the company Kraft, speak about 'childhood obesity and the growing challenge it represents for us (the processed food industry) all' (p. xvi). Mudd's simple conclusion was that these men and their industry are to blame: 'What's driving the increase (in childhood obesity)?' His answer: 'Ubiquity of inexpensive, good-tasting, super-sized, energy-dense foods' (p.xvii–xviii).

And his suggested plan of action to reverse the problem followed logically from that conclusion: 'We *are* saying that the industry should make a sincere effort to be *part* of the solution (of the childhood obesity problem). And that by doing so, we can help to defuse the criticism that's building against us. We don't have to singlehandedly *solve* the obesity problem in order to address the criticism. But we have to make a sincere effort to be *part* of the solution if we expect to avoid being demonized' (p. xx).

To do this, he suggested, the industry would have to reduce the addictive nature of the foods they produced and to stop driving overconsumption through devious advertising and marketing.

The response to Mudd's plea was direct and unambiguous. It came from Stephen Sanger then head of General Mills, a company that was then generating $2 billion a year from the sale of sugary breakfast cereals. 'Don't talk to me about nutrition. Talk to me about taste, and if this stuff tastes better, don't run around trying to sell stuff that doesn't taste good' (p. xx). And with that the processed food industry in the US turned its back on any possible role it might have in causing the global obesity and diabetes epidemics after 1980. In essence it decided that its responsibility was to generate profits. Not to worry about the health of those using its products.

In 2013, following the publication of Moss's book, the same Michael Mudd wrote an article in the *New York Times* in which he said: 'Confronted with this (claim that their industry is driving the obesity epidemic), the executives who run these companies like to say they don't create demand, they try only to satisfy it. "We're just giving people what they want. We're not putting a gun to their heads," the refrain goes. Nothing could be further from the truth. Over the years, relentless efforts were made to increase the number of "eating occasions" people indulged in and the amount of food they consumed at each'.

So there we have it. The real cause of the obesity/diabetes epidemic has little to do with a sudden global growth of sloth and gluttony. The obesity epidemic did not suddenly begin because of a massive global failure of the world's collective discipline and willpower.

Instead it is a socio-political-economic problem that began with the desire of certain US politicians in the early 1970s to ingratiate themselves with their housewives (by producing cheaper foods) and their farmers (by subsidizing the production of maize and soy). This led to the growth of the processed food industry, the profitability of which is driven by cheap, addictive, long-lived, high-carbohydrate foods that humans find irresistible.

The result is that for the first time in our 3.5 million year evolution, after 1980 humans began to eat more calories than they require for their optimal health. And as a consequence they grew fat. The only reasonable prediction is that unless there are some radical reforms, led by the world's politicians, humans will continue to grow even fatter with each succeeding generation.

Since the obesity/diabetes epidemic is a socio-political-economic problem, it cannot be solved by the medical and dietetics professions working with individual patients. It can only be solved by those governments that are prepared to legislate against industries producing those addictive foods that are driving the obesity/diabetes epidemic.

So all the world's politicians have a simple choice: Either continue to allow the unrestrained production and marketing of the processed foods that are the direct cause of the growing obesity/diabetes epidemic. In which case governments will have to invest exponentially more money in treating the medical consequences of that choice. Or promote the provision and consumption of real foods with the ultimate elimination of highly addictive processed foods. This will cause the loss of jobs and tax revenue but will dramatically improve the nation's health while reversing rising medical costs. So the money saved on sustaining a nation's ill health can be used to grow a truly healthy and productive nation.

The nations that first take this radical step will be those that dominate our collective global future.

Conclusions

The clear evidence is that it is not energy-dense high-fat foods that cause obesity even though they contain more calories (and more nutrients) than the carbohydrate-rich foods that the 1977 USDGA advised all humans to eat in order to be healthy. It is now clear that the 'experts' who gave us that advice were under undue influence from the US Government in its desire to change the nature of the foods eaten in the US and exported from there to the rest of the world. Since US scientists are more credible than those from any other country, so this advice was quickly accepted as the global 'truth' by compliant scientists elsewhere (including myself).

The decision to remove fat from the diet was not based on proven scientific evidence then available. Worse, no one asked the question: What happens when we reduce the intake of one nutrient (fat) and replace it with another (carbohydrate)? Might the solution be worse than the problem it was designed to fix?

Indeed independent scientists warned of the danger of undertaking an experiment without knowing what would be the most likely outcome. For example, Dr Philip Handler, then Director of the National Academy of Sciences, asked: 'What right has the federal government to propose that the American people conduct a vast nutritional experiment, with themselves as subjects, on the strength of so very little evidence?'

Similarly, the opinion of a leading cholesterol expert of the time, Dr Eric Ahrens, was: '... a trial of the low-fat diet recommended by the McGovern Committee and the American Heart Association has never been carried out. It seems that the proponents of this dietary change are willing to advocate an untested diet to the nation on the basis of suggestive evidence obtained in tests of a different diet. This illogic is presumably justified by the belief that benefits will be obtained, vis-à-vis CHD prevention, by any diet that causes a reduction in plasma lipid levels'.

Sadly, the results of that experiment are now all too obvious (Figure 7). The experiment failed. It is time to acknowledge the error and to start healing the world.

But if the politicians and scientists are reluctant to change, we can at least save ourselves, one person at a time, one meal at a time, by eating the real foods for which we are designed.

But won't I die from a heart attack if I eat all that fat?

This is the logical question that I am most frequently asked when I advise people that eating more fat is the healthy option.

Recall that the false idea that we should eat less, especially saturated fat, came from Ancel Keys' erroneous belief and ultimately his dogma that fat in the diet is the singular cause of heart disease. We now know that especially dietary saturated fat is unrelated to heart disease risk in individuals, as so convincingly argued by all the evidence presented in *The Big Fat Surprise* (Teicholz, 2014). Nor is there any longer any evidence that saturated fat intake predicts heart disease rates in different countries. Instead any relationship appears to be the reverse of what Keys supposedly found (Figure 4). Similarly the evidence appears to be that countries with higher blood cholesterol concentrations have lower rates of heart disease than those with lower blood cholesterol concentrations (Figures 5 and 6).

In the end Keys' failed 'plumbing model' of heart disease has proved too simple to be true. For example, his explanation is that saturated fat in the diet is converted directly into 'cholesterol' in the bloodstream, which then passively 'clogs' the arteries just as might a drainpipe become 'clogged' after years of continual use. But human arteries are not inanimate pipes. Nor is it plausible that a substance (cholesterol) is produced by our livers with the sole purpose of clogging up our arteries. Human biology simply does not work that way. If cholesterol is produced by the liver and transported in the blood to all the cells of the body, it is because it must serve an important purpose. Indeed cholesterol is one of the most critical chemicals in the body and humans could not survive without it. Without cholesterol, human life is impossible. To provide its life-sustaining actions, cholesterol is transported to all the body's cells to supplement the cholesterol that each produces for its survival. The idea that to be healthy we need to block the production of cholesterol in all our cells is perhaps the most ridiculous medical idea since blood-letting became an accepted medical practice more than 2,000 years ago. As British nutritionist Zoë Harcombe has written: 'Your liver makes cholesterol not because your liver wants you dead but because life isn't possible without cholesterol'.

The first challenge to Keys' theory arose when early epidemiological studies showed that those with higher concentrations of one form of cholesterol, HDL-cholesterol, had a lower, not a higher risk of developing heart disease. This was a disturbing finding.

But the 'experts' soon came up with a simple explanation. From henceforth cholesterol would be classified as either 'good' or 'bad'. While HDL-cholesterol may be 'good', the other major 'cholesterol' constituent, LDL-cholesterol, must be 'bad'. According to this simplistic interpretation, 'artery-clogging' LDL-cholesterol is the 'bad' form in which cholesterol is produced by the liver and then transported to the arteries, where it is free to do its 'artery-clogging' damage. In contrast the 'good' HDL-cholesterol removes some of the cholesterol from the arteries and returns it to the liver (where it can immediately be turned back into 'artery-clogging' LDL-cholesterol to be returned to the arteries in order to repeat the endless process of arterial damage and disease promotion). The illogic of this explanation of how HDL-cholesterol can be 'good' seems to have escaped the attention of those who prefer this explanation.

But cholesterol is neither 'good' nor 'bad'. It is just cholesterol. And anyone who continues to use this simplistic terminology exposes his or her ignorance of how 'cholesterol' is or is not involved in causing heart disease. When anyone uses these terms in your presence, my advice is that you absent yourself since nothing constructive will come from that ignorant discussion.

For the truth is that cholesterol does not even exist in the blood as a fat, that is as cholesterol. Instead cholesterol is insoluble in water (and blood) because it is a fat. So it can be transported in the blood only in a water-soluble form. This is achieved by covering the cholesterol with a protein lining. In this way cholesterol in the blood is in fact a protein, not a fat. The proper technical term is that cholesterol is transported in the blood as a class of proteins known as lipoproteins. Certain lipoproteins are indeed linked to an increased risk of heart disease and so some lipoproteins are indeed 'bad'. But the simplistic focus on blood 'cholesterol' as the key risk factor for heart disease is not just wrong, it is also bad for our health. For it leads directly to the wrong conclusions of which diet is best for the prevention of heart disease. Only when we understand the contribution of the different lipoproteins to our risk of developing arterial damage and heart disease can we begin to understand which diet will ensure our optimum health and minimize our risk of developing heart disease.

In the first place it is biologically impossible for humans to convert saturated fat into 'bad' LDL-cholesterol. There is simply no biochemical pathway that allows this to happen. So Keys' explanation that saturated fat in the diet causes heart disease by increasing LDL-cholesterol production should have been thrown out as a biological impossibility already in the 1950s. Instead it continues as the dominant teaching. Which raises the question: 'Why?'

Sadly the answer is because the pharmaceutical industry determines what is taught about heart disease in medical schools. Since cholesterol-lowering (statin) drugs are one of the most profitable groups of pharmaceutical agents, so the industry has no appetite for anything other than that the simplistic 'plumbing' model of heart disease should be taught to medical students or believed by all medical doctors.

Second, the 'bad' lipoproteins as well as all the other risk factors for heart disease are affected to a far greater extent by the carbohydrate than by the fat content of the diet, regardless of how much saturated fat is ingested. To understand this we need to understand in much greater detail the way in which the risk factors for heart disease (and other chronic illnesses) interact and how they are affected by either the carbohydrate or fat content of the diet.

If bad cholesterol is not the direct cause of arterial damage and heart disease, then why is cholesterol found in diseased arteries?

The 'plumbing' model of heart disease states that 'bad' LDL-cholesterol damages arteries in direct proportion to its blood concentration; the higher the concentration, the worse the arterial disease. According to this explanation 'bad' LDL-cholesterol simply crosses into the arteries when its blood concentration rises above some critical value – usually above 2–3 mmol/L.

But there are a number of logical flaws with this simple explanation. First, arteries are naturally impervious to the entry of cholesterol. Second, human arterial disease is highly selective; it occurs typically only in short sections of the (damaged) arteries and never affects veins, which constitute a major portion of the vessels in the human circulation. This shows that something other than simply the blood cholesterol concentration determines whether human blood vessels will or will not be damaged by cholesterol.

Third, the majority of persons who develop heart disease in countries like the US have blood LDL-cholesterol levels below the cut-off value considered to predict freedom from heart disease risk. Similarly the majority of persons with 'high' blood LDL-cholesterol concentrations will never suffer a heart attack.

Fourth, it has never been shown that the level of 'cholesterol' in the blood can predict the severity of disease of the coronary arteries. Thus, coronary arteries may be severely diseased in a person with total cholesterol concentrations of 3.5mmol/L but pristine in some with cholesterol levels of 9.0mmol/L. Thus, to think that one can predict the state of one's own coronary arteries simply by measuring one's blood total cholesterol concentration is naive in the extreme.

Fifth, whereas cholesterol-lowering drugs very effectively lower blood cholesterol concentrations, they are much less effective in producing long-term health benefits in those who use them. Thus new evidence shows that for one 'healthy' person with an elevated blood cholesterol concentration to benefit from taking cholesterol-lowering medication, a total of 140 persons must be treated. In a population of men with established heart disease the prediction is not much better – eighty such men must be treated for one to benefit. Do these facts really justify the spending of more than $40 billion a year on the prescription of these drugs? Similarly, in women the benefits of taking these drugs, if there are indeed any, are substantially less, requiring hundreds, perhaps thousands to be treated, for one to benefit.

Sixth is the realization that it is not the 'clogged artery' that causes heart attacks and sudden death. Rather, it is the rupture of the arterial plaque, much as an inflamed boil may burst, that causes the sudden development of a blood clot within the coronary arteries that causes

a heart attack to occur. This is at its heart an inflammatory process that is not simply due to an elevated blood cholesterol concentration. Rather, it is likely due to many factors, most of which are almost certainly due to an inflamed state within the body caused by high carbohydrate diets in those with IR.

The alternate explanation is that arteries are damaged by the entry of only one form of lipoprotein, the small, dense LDL-cholesterol particles, and then only if those small, dense LDL-cholesterol particles have been damaged by becoming oxidized. It is proposed that oxidized small, dense LDL-cholesterol particles have the ability to enter damaged arteries where they become 'stuck' within the arterial wall, inducing an inflammatory reaction that leads ultimately to the irreversible arterial damage recognized as the arterial plaque.

Thus according to the explanation it is not 'cholesterol' which causes arterial damage but rather the entry of small, dense, oxidized LDL-particles into arteries.

Since diets high in carbohydrate or fat have opposite effects on the blood concentrations of 'cholesterol' and small, dense LDL-cholesterol so the diet that appears optimum for health will be different depending on whether you believe it is 'cholesterol' or small, dense LDL-cholesterol particles that cause arterial damage and heart disease.

Importantly we need to know what factors cause arteries to become damaged and what factors lead to the oxidation of small, dense LDL-cholesterol particles.

The complete picture: Risk factors for heart disease and how they are influenced by the carbohydrate or fat content of the diet

(i) Factors predicting risk of future heart attack

The most recent (2012) analysis of the risk factors that, according to the 'plumbing' model, predict future risk for heart disease are listed below in Table 1. In that table the 'risk' factors are listed according to the relative strength of their ability to predict future risk of heart attack. For example, a Relative Risk of 2 indicates that that risk factor predicts a twofold increased risk of heart disease or a 100 per cent increase compared with a factor that added no risk and so had a Relative Risk of 1.

TABLE 1: Hazard Ratios for seven factors considered to predict future risk for the development of Coronary Heart Disease.

RISK FACTOR	HAZARD RATIO (RELATIVE RISK)
Diabetes	2.04
Age	1.87
Current Smoking	1.79
High Blood Pressure	1.31
Total Blood Cholesterol concentration	1.22
Blood Triglyceride concentration	1.19
Blood HDL-Cholesterol concentration	0.83

Of these factors, only diabetes, age and current smoking are the more powerful predictors. An elevated total blood cholesterol concentration predicts only a 22 per cent increased risk of heart disease that, according to the nature of these predictions, is almost meaningless. In fact of all the factors only one, diabetes, really stands out as a powerful predictor of heart attack risk.

It is also known that the increased risk of heart attack in diabetics is not explained by higher blood LDL-cholesterol concentrations since their values are no higher than those without diabetes who also develop heart disease. What is it about diabetes that causes heart disease?

(ii) Why do abnormalities in carbohydrate metabolism elevate the risk of arterial damage and heart disease in persons with IR and type 2 diabetes?

As I have already hinted, it is the abnormal metabolic state induced by the effects of a high carbohydrate diet which produces the toxic triad of high blood triglyceride and small dense LDL-cholesterol particles combined with low HDL-cholesterol concentrations that is especially damaging to the arteries of those with IR. Particularly when combined with continually elevated blood glucose and insulin concentrations.

It is the abnormally elevated blood glucose concentrations that explain why diabetics are at such high risk for developing arterial damage leading to heart disease.

A key finding is that the single best predictor of heart attack risk is the blood concentration of glycosylated haemoglobin (HbA1c). The blood HbA1c concentration is a measure of the average blood glucose concentration over the previous twelve weeks. It is an indicator of the extent to which elevated blood glucose concentrations have damaged key body proteins by adding glucose (glycosylation) to any proteins in direct contact with the blood. Glycosylation alters protein function, making them less effective in their various functions. Since haemoglobin is one of the most abundant proteins in blood, the extent to which it is glycosylated gives a good indication of the extent to which other critical body proteins have been damaged by too-high blood glucose concentrations.

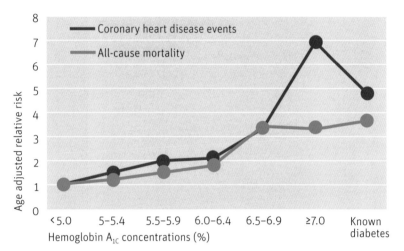

FIGURE 12: Age-adjusted relative risk of developing coronary heart disease rises as a function of the blood HbA1c concentration. Note that relative risk begins to rise steeply above an HbA1c concentration of 6.4 and is increased sevenfold in those with an HbA1c greater than 7 per cent. This compares with an increase in relative risk of only 1.2 in those with 'elevated' blood cholesterol concentrations (Table 1, opposite). (From Khaw et al. 2004.)

Ischaemic heart disease

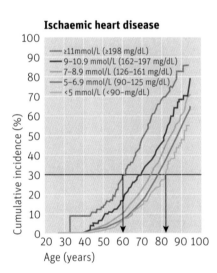

Heart attack (Myocardial infarction)

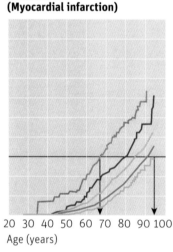

FIGURE 13: Cumulative incidence of diagnoses of ischaemic heart disease (left panel) and of heart attacks (right panel) in persons with different blood glucose concentrations measured at random. Note that risk rises at any increasing level of blood glucose concentration. The HCLF diet increases and the LCHF Diet reduces random blood glucose concentrations (Figure 5). (From Benn et al. 2012.)

Figure 12 shows how the Relative Risk for coronary heart disease events including heart attacks and for deaths from all-causes (all-cause mortality) rises with increasing blood HbA1c concentrations. Note that HbA1c values above 6.4 per cent are associated with a sudden exponential increase in risk for heart disease and all-cause mortality so that an HbA1c value in excess of 7 per cent is associated with a sevenfold higher risk for a coronary heart disease event. Compare this to the 1.22-fold increased risk for heart disease event if one has a 'high' blood cholesterol concentration (Table 1).

Another study reported the cumulative incidence (per cent) of coronary heart disease (Figure 13, left) and of heart attacks (Figure 13, right) as a function of a random blood glucose concentration measured at any time during the day. It shows that by the age of sixty, 30 per cent of those with random blood glucose concentrations greater than 11mol/L (indicating the presence of type 2 diabetes) had already been diagnosed with coronary heart disease. Whereas only by the age of eighty had the same percentage of those with a random blood glucose concentration below 5mmol/L received the same diagnosis. The right panel of Figure 13 shows that by age ninety-three only 30 per cent of those with a blood glucose concentration below 5mmol/L had suffered a heart attack whereas already by age sixty-eight, 30 per cent of those with blood glucose concentrations greater than 11mmol/L had suffered the same fate.

This evidence suggests that high blood glucose concentrations are the single most important factor predicting risk that arterial damage causing heart disease will develop. It seems that glucose damages arteries directly through the glycosylation effect on key proteins and also by promoting oxidation of the small dense LDL-cholesterol particles.

Another piece of the puzzle comes from the same study showing the ability of elevated HbA1c concentrations to predict future heart attack risk. That study also included two other measures of blood fat concentrations, blood HDL-cholesterol and blood triglyceride concentrations (Figure 14). Those data showed that subsequent mortality over the twelve years of follow-up in the study in both men (left panel) and women (right panel) was least in those who had a combination of high blood HDL-cholesterol concentrations and low blood triglyceride concentrations (top lines) and was worst (bottom lines) in those with the opposite – low blood concentrations of 'good' HDL-cholesterol and high blood triglyceride concentrations.

The factors linking these findings are the following: high-carbohydrate diets in those with IR cause elevated blood glucose concentrations and high HbA1c concentrations leading ultimately to type 2 diabetes. But high-carbohydrate diets also cause elevated blood

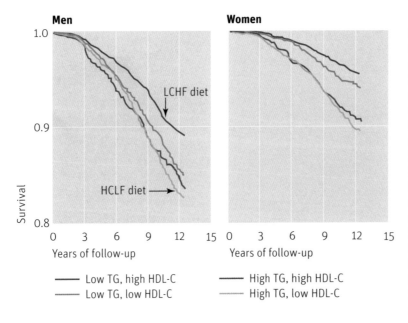

FIGURE 14: Survival curves for individuals with either of four different combinations of blood HDL-cholesterol and triglyceride concentrations in men (left panel) and women (right panel). Note that the greatest survival (upper curves in both panels) occurs in those who have a combination of high blood HDL-cholesterol and low triglyceride concentrations whereas the worst survival (lowest curves in both panels) occurs in those with the opposite – low blood HDL-cholesterol and high blood triglyceride concentrations. Interestingly, the LCHF Diet produces the former (favourable) combination whereas the HCLF Diet produces the unfavourable combination of low blood HDL-cholesterol and high triglyceride concentrations especially in those who are the most insulin resistant. (From Rana et al. 2010.)

triglyceride concentrations and lower HDL-cholesterol concentrations in those with IR.

Thus the common factor linking these findings are high-carbohydrate diets in those with IR/type 2 diabetes.

(iii) The studies of Drs Jeff Volek, Stephen Phinney and Eric Westman show that all risk factors improve on a low-carbohydrate diet.

Recall that Dr Robert Atkins, MD began to fund the research of Drs Volek, Phinney and Westman shortly before his death. The result is a body of novel information best captured in their excellent books *The New Atkins for a New You, The Art and Science of Low Carbohydrate Living* and *The Art and Science of Low Carbohydrate Performance*. The results of one of their best studies is shown in Figure 15, below, which compares changes in a number of blood and other predictors of health in two groups of

matched obese subjects who were placed on a reduced calorie HCLF or LCHF Diet while their responses were carefully measured.

The results showed that in all these key variables, subjects on Banting showed more advantageous changes than did those assigned to the supposedly more healthy HCLF Diet. It is important to note that on the LCHF Diet, all risk factors moved in the same direction – that is all improved and the degree of improvement was substantially more than were changes in those following the HCLF Diet.

Thus besides greater reductions in body weight and blood pressure, there were greater reductions in parameters of abnormal glucose metabolism, in blood triglyceride and VLDL-cholesterol concentrations (another form of 'bad' cholesterol), and small dense LDL-cholesterol particle numbers whereas the blood concentration of the 'good' HDL-cholesterol

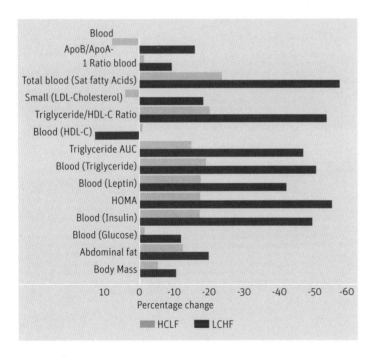

FIGURE 15: The study of Volek et al. (2008) showed that subjects who lost weight on the LCHF Diet showed greater changes in all measured coronary risk factors than did those eating a hypocaloric HCLF Diet. Key: [ ] = concentration; AUC = Area Under the Curve; HOMA = Homeostasis Model Assessment; Sat = Saturated. Note that the LCHF reduces, whereas the HCLF Diet increases the number of small, dense LDL-cholesterol particles that are associated with arterial damage. Total blood saturated fats also fall more on the LCHF than on the HCLF Diet. Only the LCHF increases blood HDL-cholesterol concentrations and reduces the blood ApoB/ApoA-1 ratio.

TABLE 2: *Risk factors for the development of arterial damage and Coronary Heart Disease*

	RISK FACTOR	TEST	IDEAL READING	THRESHOLD
MARKERS OF ABNORMAL CARBOHYDRATE METABOLISM	Body Weight/Body Mass Index/% Body Fat	BMI test	<25 kg/m^2	>25 kg/m2
	Blood Pressure	Blood Pressure Tested – rest for 15 minutes first	110 – 130/65 – 80 mmHg	140/85 max mmHg
	Blood Glucose concentration	Standard Blood Test (After a 12 hour fast)	<5 mmol/L	>5.5 mmol/L
	Blood Insulin concentration	Standard Blood Test (After a 12 hour fast)	<5µU/ml	>9µU/ml
	Blood Glucose Tolerance Test (with measurement of insulin concentrations)	If suspected diabetic	2-hour blood glucose concentration <7.8 mmol/L	2-hour blood concentration >7.8 mmol/L
	Blood HbA1c concentration	Standard Blood Test (After a 12 hour fast)	<5%	>6.5%
	Blood Ketone Body concentration	Ketostick test	0.5 mmol/L	>0.5 mmol/L
	Blood HDL-Cholesterol concentration	Standard Blood Test (After a 12 hour fast)	Male >2 and Women >2 mmol/L	Male <1.2 Women <1.7 mmol/L
	Blood Triglyceride concentration – NB	Standard Blood Test (After a 12 hour fast)	<1 mmol/L	>1.7 mmol/L
	Blood Uric Acid concentration	Standard Blood Test (After a 12 hour fast)	<360µmol/L Females <420µmol/L Males	>360µmol/L Females >420µmol/L Males
	Presence of Non-Alcoholic Fatty Liver on ultrasound	Ultrasound Test	No evidence of fatty liver	Presence of fatty liver
ABNORMAL LIPOPROTEINS	Blood concentration and number of small LDL-Cholesterol particles	Standard blood test	Pattern A: low number of small LDL-particles	Pattern B: increased number of small LDL-particles
	Blood Apo-B concentration	Standard blood test	<90 mg/dL <17 x 10^{-4} mMol/L	<90 mg/dL <17 x 10^{-4} mMol/L

	HDL/Triglyceride Ratio (mmol/L)	Standard blood test (after a 12-hour fast)	<0.87	>1.74
MARKERS OF INFLAMMATION	Blood ultrasensitive CRP concentration	Standard Blood Test (After a 12 hour fast)	<1 mg/L is low risk 0.3 mg/L to 0.5mg/L is ideal	>3 mg/L is increased risk
	Blood or Tissue omega-6/omega-3 ratio	EPA/AA reading (expensive)	1:1	4:1
OTHERS	Blood Homocysteine concentration	Standard blood test	4–15 micromoles/L	>15 micromoles/L
	Blood Fibrinogen concentration – Clotting factor	Standard blood test	150–250 mg/dL	>250 mg/dL

concentrations also increased more on the LCHF diet. This occurred without significant increases in 'bad' LDL-cholesterol concentrations.

Instead if LDL-cholesterol concentrations rise in those eating the LCHF, this is due to an increase in the concentration of the large LDL-cholesterol particles which are not harmful as they can neither be oxidized, nor do they 'stick' inside the arterial wall. Thus they do not contribute to the development of the arterial plaque that is the key pathological abnormality in the arterial damage that leads to coronary heart disease.

In contrast, ingestion of a HCLF Diet increases fat production in the liver (hepatic de novo lipogenesis – itself a risk factor for arterial damage – Table 2), which raises blood triglyceride concentrations and lowers blood HDL-cholesterol concentrations. These responses, the opposite of those occurring in response to the Banting Diet, are considered to promote arterial damage and are associated with a reduced long-term survival (Figure 14).

The evidence that Banting produced the greatest benefits in those who are the most ill is in line with all this evidence and neatly destroys the prejudice that a high-fat diet is a dangerous 'fad'. Instead the logical conclusion must be that Banting is the safer option for those who are the most ill because they have morbid obesity, diabetes, hypertension and hypercholesterolaemia as a result of more severe IR.

Thus all this evidence suggests that the 'healthy' HCLF Diet will be much less effective in preventing future heart attacks than is Banting and most especially in those with more severe degrees of IR.

Which is in line with the evidence that humans were much healthier in the past while Banting than they are today eating the 'heart-healthy' HCLF Diet.

(iv) So, it's not just 'good' and 'bad' cholesterol

The finding that the risk factors for heart disease measured by Volek, Phinney and Westman all improved on Banting suggests that we should rather consider risk factors for heart disease as a collective, not simply in terms of either 'good' or

TABLE 3 *indicates the values that are optimal for long-term health and the effects of low-carb and low-fat diets on these variables.*

VARIABLE	WHAT IT SHOULD BE	WHAT A LOW-CARB DIET DOES	WHAT A LOW-FAT HIGH-CARBOHYDRATE DIET DOES IN THOSE WITH IR OR MS
Body weight	What it was as 20-year-old	Reduces	Increases
Blood pressure	Low – below 125/75mmHg	Reduces	Increases
Blood fasting glucose concentration	Low – below 5.0mmol/L	Reduces	Increases
Blood fasting insulin concentration	Low – below 5µU/ml	Reduces	Increases
Blood glycated haemoglobin (%)	Below 5.5%	Reduces	Increases
Blood triglyceride concentration	Below 0.75mmol/L	Reduces	Increases
Blood HDL-cholesterol concentration	Above 2.0mmol/L	Raises	Lowers
Number of small dense LDL particles in blood	Low	Reduces	Increases
Number of large fluffy LDL particles	Most of the LDL-cholesterol should be in these particles	Raises	Lowers
Total number of LDL-cholesterol particles in blood	Low	Unknown	Increases
Blood apoB concentration	Low	Reduces	Increases

'bad' cholesterol. Table 2 lists all the important factors that have been identified as predicting risk of future heart attack. I have listed them as markers of abnormal carbohydrate metabolism, abnormal lipoproteins, markers of inflammation and others.

The point is that these measures give a true indicator of one's real risk of heart disease in a way that the simple measurement of the blood concentrations of 'good' and 'bad' cholesterol is quite unable. Importantly, if many or most of these variables are abnormal, it indicates the presence of greater levels of IR and hence an even greater urgency to adopt the LCHF eating plan as a matter of extreme priority. Recall from Figure 1 that IR is the most frequent but overlooked common cause for obesity, diabetes, hypertension (high blood pressure) and perhaps elevated blood cholesterol concentrations (hypercholesterolaemia).

The practical point is that if one wants to understand properly what is one's real risk for developing heart disease sometime in the future, then these are the variables that need to be measured.

The greater the number of normal results, the lower is one's risk. For the reason that the fewer abnormalities that are detected, the lesser the degree of IR, which is the real driver of abnormalities in all these tests.

On the other hand the greater the number of abnormal tests, the greater the degree of IR and the greater the need to reduce the number of grams of carbohydrate eaten to an absolute minimum, preferably less than 50 g/day, as discussed in the following section.

It is not just about heart disease

Type 2 diabetes mellitus does not increase only one's risk for developing arterial damage and coronary heart disease. Instead those with type 2 diabetes are also at greatly increased risk of the development of cancer and dementias like Alzheimer's disease. Is it possible that chronically elevated blood glucose concentrations might also promote those diseases?

The answer is almost certainly yes. For example, a recent study found that elevated blood glucose concentrations were a predictor for risk of dementia in both those with and without type 2 diabetes so that the higher the average blood glucose concentration, the greater the risk of dementia. Thus the message: If you want to protect your brain, you need to keep your blood glucose concentration down.

Then there is growing evidence that the key abnormality in cancer is an increased capacity to utilize glucose. In fact, cancer cells do not have the capacity to use any fuel for their growth other than glucose. Unlike the humans in which they occur, cancer cells have an absolute requirement for glucose. Without glucose they starve to death, a point first realized by Dr Otto Warburg, who won the 1931 Nobel Prize for discovering this phenomenon.

Thus the certainty that because they promote the overconsumption of carbohydrates, the 1977 USDGA must also have contributed to the growing incidence of cancer and dementia since 1977.

Taking to Banting

The key prediction of the 'Yudkin Paradox' and the reason why the Banting Diet is so effective is because it focuses on limiting the carbohydrate content of the diet. Since it is the carbohydrate content that drives hunger and so determines how many calories must be eaten to produce satiation, so Banting must also be the most effective method of weight loss. In contrast, eating a low-calorie HCLF Diet cannot work in the majority since this dietary pattern will induce hunger, not sustainable weight loss.

In addition, those with IR must restrict their grams of carbohydrate eaten every day in order to lower their blood insulin concentrations, to allow fat to be released from their fat cells and so used as a fuel. Continuing to eat more than a limited amount of carbohydrates keeps insulin concentrations high and so prevents weight loss. What many obese fail to appreciate perhaps is just how few grams of carbohydrate those with severe IR may ingest if they are to remain lean.

To explain this concept I have designed a unique, never-seen-before figure (Figure 16), which proposes that the key drivers of one's Body Mass Index (BMI) are the average number of grams of carbohydrate eaten each day and the extent of each individual's IR. This is a conceptual slide – it is not yet based on measured data but is used to explain what appears to be the truth.

What Figure 16 aims to show is that persons with extreme insulin sensitivity – the opposite to IR – can eat as many grams of carbohydrate each day as they wish without ever becoming fat. In this theoretical model someone with extreme insulin sensitivity would be able to eat up to 500 g per day of carbohydrate (left edge of diagram) – about two and a half times what I think is necessary – while retaining a BMI

at the bottom of the normal range. Most elite endurance athletes are probably in this group.

A person with mild IR would be able to eat perhaps up to 250 g of carbohydrate per day while also maintaining a low BMI. But at higher intakes he or she might show a progressive increase in BMI. As a result a person with this level of IR would still be able to sustain a healthy BMI less than 25kg/m2 even when eating 400 g/day of carbohydrate.

Similarly, individuals with moderate IR would be able to regulate their weight within the safe range at carbohydrate intakes of up to 200 g/day. But above that intake their BMI would increase more steeply so that at intakes greater than about 300 g/day they would no longer be able to control their BMI in the safe range and at an intake of 500 g/day they might even reach an obese BMI.

Those who are markedly IR might be able to maintain a normal BMI of less than 25 kg/m2 when eating less than about 175 g carbohydrate/day. At higher intakes they would rapidly develop BMIs rated as either overweight or obese.

Finally, those with severe and morbid IR are perhaps able to maintain a healthy BMI only on a miniscule amount of daily carbohydrate, perhaps less than about 25–50 g/day. Once they exceed that threshold, their BMI rises steeply so that eating as little as 200 g/day will cause them to have a BMI in excess of 25–30 kg/m2 respectively, classifying them as either overweight or obese class 1.

It is utterly critical to understand that range in the number of grams of carbohydrate that each of us can eat in order to maintain a healthy BMI narrows with increasing levels of IR. Thus persons with morbid IR can eat only within a range of 0–25 g carbs per day if they wish

Different carbohydrate intakes in insulin resistance (IR)

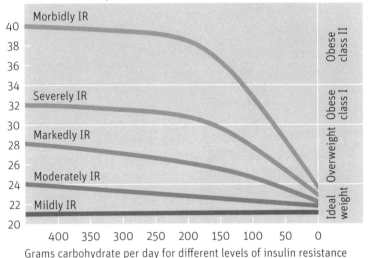

FIGURE 16: A concept figure showing the postulated relationship between the amount of carbohydrates eaten each day and the Body Mass Index (BMI) in individuals with different degrees of insulin resistance (IR). Note that those with increasing IR have higher BMI at any given level of daily carbohydrate intake so those who are morbidly insulin resistant must cut their daily carbohydrate intake to about 25–50 g/day if they are ever to maintain a BMI less than 25 kg/m2.

to be lean. The slightest increase above that range will rapidly cause weight gain in part because hunger returns and with it the urge to eat more carbohydrate calories. This explains why traditional dietary advice which allows 'everything in moderation' fails spectacularly in those with IR. Because there is no 'moderate' carbohydrate intake that will allow those with morbid IR to remain lean. For them, only extreme measures will ever work.

According to the diagram above the amount of carbohydrate each of us can eat each day is determined by our individual level of IR. As a result the key to maintaining our long-term health is, in my opinion, to maintain a BMI of 25 kg/m2 or less by eating only the number of grams of carbohydrate/day that will allow an ideal BMI for our individual levels of IR. There is still much work to be done on the brain regulation of hunger and calorie consumption in those who do spectacularly well. Table 3 gives some of the ideal blood readings, all of which also improve in those with IR who reduce their daily carbohydrate intake to the ideal amount (Figure 16).

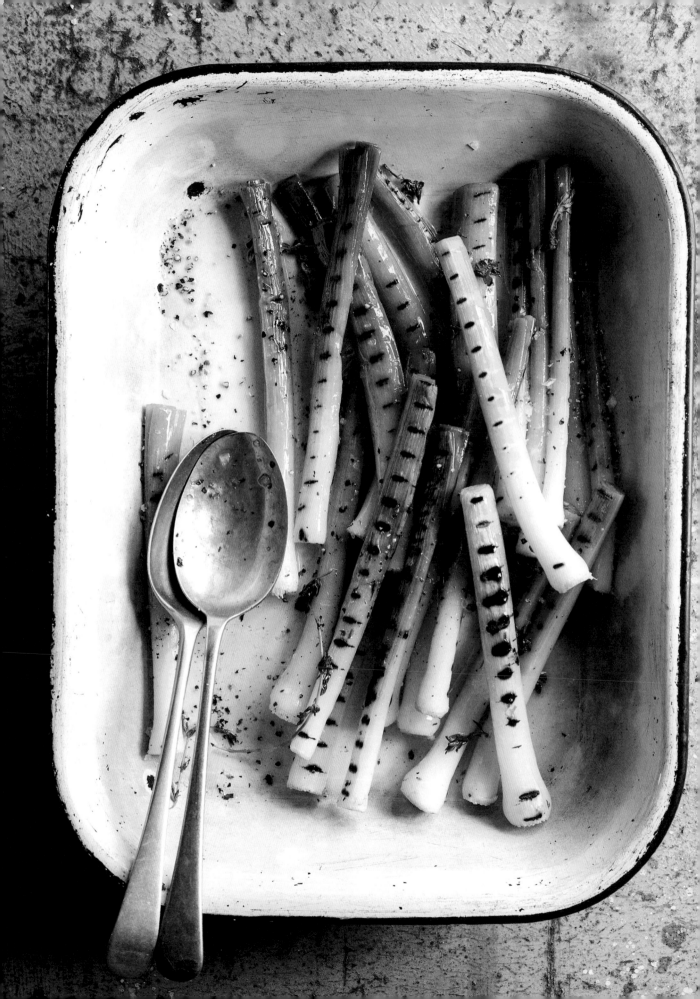

BIBLIOGRAPHY

Ajala, O., English, P., Pinkney, J., 'Systematic review and meta-analysis of different dietary approaches to the management of type 2 diabetes' (Am J Clin Nutr 2013) 97(3):505–516.

Anonymous, 'The Swedes are eating more butter!' (eBlogger 2009). http://lowcarb4u. blogspot.com/2009/06/swedes-are-eating-more-butter.html.

Atkins R. C., *Dr Atkins Diet Revolution* 1st ed. (New York: David McKay Company, Inc., 1972) 1–310.

Banting, W., *Letter of Corpulence* 3rd edition, (San Francisco: A. Roman & Co., 1865) 1–64.

Bauer, J., *Obesity: Its pathogenesis, etiology and treatment* (Arch Intern Med 1941) 67(5) 968–994.

Brillat-Savarin J. A., *The Physiology of Taste* ebooks@Adelaide, (2012). http://ebooks. adelaide.edu.au/b/brillat/savarin/b85p.

Brillat-Savarin J. A., Simpson L. F., *The Handbook of Dining: Or how to dine theoretically, philosophically and historically considered* (London: Longman, Brown, Green, Longmans & Roberts, 1859) 1–244.

Bueno, N. B., de Melo, I. S., de Oliveira, S.L., da Rocha, A. T., 'Very-low-carbohydrate ketogenic diet v. low-fat diet for long-term weight loss: a meta-analysis of randomised controlled trials' (*British Journal of Nutrition* 2013) Epub:1–10.

Catsicas, R., *The complete nutritional solution to diabetes* (Cape Town, SA: Random House Struik, 2009) 1–192.

Coulston, A. M., Hollenbeck, C. B., Swislocki, A. L., Chen, Y. D., Reaven, G. M., 'Deleterious metabolic effects of high-carbohydrate, sucrose-containing diets in patients with non-insulin-dependent diabetes mellitus' (Am J Med 1987) 82(2):213-220.

De Wet, N., 'Are we ready to explore the use of low carbohydrate diets in the nutritional management of obesity and Type 2 diabetes?' (SA J Diabetes 2012) Aug:11–16.

Dukan, P., *The Dukan Diet* (London: Hodder & Stoughton, 2010) 1–384.

Ebstein W., *Fettleibigkeit (Corpulenz)* (Wiesbaden: J. F. Bergmann, 1883) 1–54.

Ebstein, W., 'Corpulence and its treatment on physiological principles'. (Translated by Keane, A. H., London, Covent Garden, H. Grevel, 1884.)

Falta, W., *Endocrine diseases, including their diagnosis and treatment.* 3rd ed. (London: J. & A. Churchill, 1923) 1-669.

Feinman, R. D., 'Fad diets in the treatment of diabetes' (Curr Diab Rep 2011) 11(2):128–135.

Gardner, C. D., Kiazand, A., Alhassan, S., et al., 'Comparison of the Atkins, Zone, Ornish, and LEARN diets for change in weight and related risk factors among overweight premenopausal women: the A to Z Weight Loss Study: a randomized trial' (JAMA 2007) 297(9):969–977.

Goodpaster, B. H., Delany, J. P., Otto, A. D., et al., 'Effects of diet and physical activity interventions on weight loss and cardiometabolic risk factors in severely obese adults: a randomized trial' (JAMA 2010) 304(16):1795–1802. [PMC3082279]

Harvey, W., 'On corpulence in relation to disease: With some remarks on diet (1872)' (London: Henry Renshaw, 1872) 1–148.

Health Professions Council of South Africa, Guidelines for good practice in the health care professions: Ethical and professional rules of the Health Professions Council of South Africa as promulgated in the Government Gazette R717/2006. HPCSA 2008. http://www.hpcsa.co.za/downloads/conduct_ethics/rules/generic_ethical_rules/booklet_2_generic_ethical_rules_with_anexures.pdf.

Heshka, S., Anderson, J. W., Atkinson, R. L., et al., 'Weight loss with self-help compared with a structured commercial program: a randomized trial' (JAMA 2003) 289(14):1792–1798.

Hooper L., Abdelhamid A., Moore H. J., et al., 'Effect of reducing total fat intake on body weight: systematic review and meta-analysis of randomised controlled trials and cohort studies' (BMJ 2012) 345:e7666. [PMC3516671]

Hu, T., Mills, K. T., Yao, L., et al. 'Effects of low-carbohydrate diets versus low-fat diets on metabolic risk factors: a meta-analysis of randomized controlled clinical trials' (Am J Epidemiol 2012) 176 Suppl 7:S44–S54. [PMC3530364]

Hussain, T. A., Mathew, T. C., Dashti, A. A., et al., 'Effect of low-calorie versus low-carbohydrate ketogenic diet in type 2 diabetes' (Nutrition 2012) 28(10):1016-1021.

Joslin, E. P., 'Pathology of diabetes mellitus' (Lecture to the Boylston Medical Society of the Harvard Medical School 1893).

Joslin, E. P., 'A diabetic manual for the mutual use of doctor and patient' (Philadelphia: Lea & Febiger, 1919) 1–192.

Krauss, R. M., Blanche, P. J., Rawlings, R. S., Fernstrom, H. S., Williams, P. T., 'Separate effects of reduced carbohydrate intake and weight loss on atherogenic dyslipidemia' (Am J Clin Nutr 2006) 83(5):1025–1031.

Lennerz, B. S., Alsop, D. C., Holsen, L. M., et al., 'Effects of dietary glycemic index on brain regions related to reward and craving in men' (Am J Clin Nutr, 2013).

Mackarness, R., Eat Fat and Grow Slim (London: The Harvill Press, 1958) 1–128.

McClellan W. S., Du Bois E. F., Prolonged meat diets with a study of kidney function and ketosis. (J Biol Chem 1930) XLV 651–667.

Newburgh L. H., Johnston, M. W., 'The Nature of Obesity' (J Clin Invest 1930) 8(2) 197–213. [PMC424616]

Noakes, T. D., Vlismas, M. Challenging Beliefs: Memoirs of a career 2nd ed. (Cape Town: Zebra Press, 2012) 1–392.

Noakes, T. D., 'Tim Noakes on Carbohydrates'. Health 24 2013. http://www.health24.com/Diet-and-nutrition/Nutrition-basics/Tim-Noakes-on-carbohydrates-20120721.

Nordmann, A. J., Nordmann, A., Briel, M., et al. 'Effects of low-carbohydrate vs low-fat diets on weight loss and cardiovascular risk factors: a meta-analysis of randomized controlled trials' (Arch Intern Med 2006) 166(3):285–293.

Osler, W., The principles and practice of medicine (New York: D. Appleton and Company, 1978) 2–1079.

Paoli, A., Rubini, A., Volek, J. S., Grimaldi, K. A., 'Beyond weight loss: a review of the therapeutic uses of very-low-carbohydrate (ketogenic) diets' (Eur J Clin Nutr 2013).

Petersen, K.F., Dufour, S., Savage, D. B., et al., 'The role of skeletal muscle insulin resistance in the pathogenesis of the metabolic syndrome' (Proc Natl Acad Sci U S A 2007) 104(31):12587–12594. [PMC1924794]

Roberts, R., Bickerton, A. S., Fielding, B. A., et al., 'Reduced oxidation of dietary fat after a short term high-carbohydrate diet' (Am J Clin Nutr 2008) 87(4):824–831.

Santos, F. L., Esteves, S. S., da Costa, P. A., Yancy, W. S., Jr., Nunes, J. P., 'Systematic review and meta-analysis of clinical trials of the effects of low carbohydrate diets on cardiovascular risk factors' (Obes Rev 2012) 13(11):1048–1066.

Schwarz, J. M., Linfoot, P., Dare, D., 'Aghajanian K. Hepatic de novo lipogenesis in normoinsulinemic and hyperinsulinemic subjects consuming high-fat, low-carbohydrate and low-fat, high-carbohydrate isoenergetic diets' (Am J Clin Nutr 2003) 77(1):43–50.

Smith, G. C., Pell, J. P., 'Parachute use to prevent death and major trauma related to gravitational challenge: systematic review of randomised controlled trials' (BMJ 2003) 327(7429) 1459-1461. [PMC300808]

Stefansson V., The Friendly Arctic (New York: The Macmillan Company, 1921) 1–898.

Stefansson, V., The Fat of the Land (New York: The MacMillan Company, 1956) 1–339.

Stock, A. L., Yudkin, J., 'Nutrient intake of subjects on low carbohydrate diet used in treatment of obesity' (Am J Clin Nutr 1970) 23(7):948–952.

Taubes, G., Why we get fat and what to do about it (New York: Knopf of Random House, 2011) 1–257.

Taubes, G., Good Calories, Bad Calories (New York: Anchor Books, 2007) 1–609.

Taubes, G., 'The science of obesity: what do we really know about what makes us fat? An essay by Gary Taubes' (BMJ 2013) 346:13.

Thompson, V., Eat and Grow Thin (New York: Cosimo Classics, 2005) 1–104.

Volek, J. S., Fernandez, M. L., Feinman, R. D., Phinney, S. D., 'Dietary carbohydrate restriction induces a unique metabolic state positively affecting atherogenic dyslipidemia, fatty acid partitioning, and metabolic syndrome' (Prog Lipid Res 2008) 47(5):307–318.

Volek, J. S., Phinney, S. D., Forsythe, C. E., et al. 'Carbohydrate restriction has a more favorable impact on the metabolic syndrome than a low fat diet' (Lipids 2009) 44(4):297–309.

Volek, J. S., Phinney, S. D., 'A New Look at Carbohydrate-Restricted Diets: Separating Fact From Fiction' (Nutrition Today 2013) 48(2):E1–E7.

Von Noorden, C., 'Obesity'. In: Von Noorden, C, Hall, I. W. (eds.) 'Metabolism and practical medicine' (Keener, 1907) 693–715.

Westman, E. C., Yancy, W. S., Jr., Olsen, M. K., Dudley, T., Guyton, J. R., 'Effect of a low-carbohydrate, ketogenic diet program compared to a low-fat diet on fasting lipoprotein subclasses' (Int J Cardiol 2006) 110(2):212–216.

Westman, E. C., Yancy, W. S., Jr., Humphreys, M, 'Dietary treatment of diabetes mellitus in the pre-insulin era (1914–1922) (Perspect Biol Med 2006) 49(1):77–83.

Yudkin, J., Carey, M., 'The treatment of obesity by the "high fat" diet. The inevitability of calories' (Lancet 1960) 2(7157):939–941.

Yudkin, J., This slimming business (Middlesex, UK: Penguin Books Ltd, 1971) 1–208.

GENERAL INDEX

Page numbers in *italic* refer to Figures.

polyunsaturated oils 254
Price, Dr Weston 266
processed foods 249, 250, 267, 276, 277, 278
    addictive potential 272, 276, 277
protein, dietary 247, 248, 257, 261, 271, 274
protein-calorie malnutrition 248
proteins 249, 280

R

Reaven, Dr Gerald 274

S

Sanger, Stephen 277
saturated fat 252, 253, 254, 255, 256,
    257, 262, 279, 280
smoking 253, *253*, 282
statin drugs 256, 280, 281
Stefansson, Vilhjalmur 262
Stock, Dr Anne 265
stroke 259
sugar 254, 256, 262, 272, 275, 276
sweating 246–7

T

Taubes, Gary 271–2
Teicholz, Nina 251, 258
trans-fats 254
triglycerides 274, 282, 284, 285, 286, 287, 288

U

uric acid 286

V

vegetable oils 254, 256
visceral adiposity 274
Volek, Dr Jeff 262, 272, 285

W

Warburg, Dr Otto 289
Westman, Dr Eric 262, 285
Women's Health Initiative Randomized
    Controlled Dietary Modification Trial
    (WHIRCDMT) 258–9

Y

Yerushalmy, Dr 254
Yudkin, Professor John 253, 254, 264
'Yudkin paradox' 264–5, 290

INDEX OF RECIPES

CONVERSION TABLES

WEIGHT

Metric	Imperial
25 g	1 oz
50 g	2 oz
75 g	3 oz
100 g	4 oz
150 g	5 oz
175 g	6 oz
200 g	7 oz
225 g	8 oz
250 g	9 oz
300 g	10 oz
325 g	11 oz
350 g	12 oz
375 g	13 oz
400 g	14 oz
450 g	1 lb

VOLUME

Metric	Imperial	US cup
5 ml	1 tsp	1 tsp
15 ml	1 tbsp	1 tbsp
50 ml	2 fl oz	3 tbsp
60 ml	2½ fl oz	4 tbsp
75 ml	3 fl oz	⅓ cup
100 ml	4 fl oz	scant ½ cup
125 ml	4 fl oz	½ cup
150 ml	5 fl oz	⅔ cup
200 ml	7 fl oz	scant 1 cup
250 ml	10 fl oz	1 cup
300 ml	½ pint	1¼ cups
350 ml	12 fl oz	1⅓ cups
450 ml	¾ pint	1¾ cups
500 ml	20 fl oz	2 cups
600 ml	1 pint	2½ cups

MEASUREMENTS

Metric	Imperial
1 cm	½ in
2 cm	¾ in
4 cm	1½ in
5 cm	2 in
10 cm	4 in
12 cm	4½ in

Metric	Imperial
13 cm	5 in
15 cm	6 in
18 cm	7 in
20 cm	8 in
25 cm	10 in
30 cm	12 in